COMPASSIONATE SNOB

WASHING OFF THE FAKE

What life taught me while surviving a brain hemorrhage

SHERI THOMPSON MCINTYRE

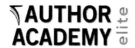

AUTHOR ACADEMY elite

Printed in the United States of America
Published by Author Academy Elite
P.O. Box 43, Powell, OH 43035

www.AuthorAcademyElite.com

Title: Compassionate Snob: Washing Off the Fake
What life taught me while surviving a brain hemorrhage

Paperback: 978-1-64085-379-9
Hardback: 978-1-64085-380-5
Ebook: 978-1-64085-381-2
Library of Congress Control Number: 201895277

Endorsements

Compassionate Snob is a head-on account of the trials and tribulations of a brain injury survivor in her recovery. This is a must-read for any aneurysm, or other brain injury patient, their caregivers and friends. One can only hope that each reader will stop and THINK as Sheri so eloquently asks we do."

Christine Buckley, Executive Director -
The Brain Aneurysm Foundation website:
https://www.bafound.org/

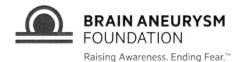

BRAIN ANEURYSM
FOUNDATION
Raising Awareness. Ending Fear.™

This book is dedicated to:
Billy and Madison,
My Sister Laurie,
My Parents
Family and Friends
The Doctors, and Nurses, and the Medical team

I wouldn't be here without you!
But most of all this book is dedicated to all the people that have
been afflicted by a brain AVM (arteriovenous malformation)
Aneurysm and TBI (Traumatic Brain Injury) etc… You are all
fighting a battle every single day. You are true warriors!

Contents

Foreword

My sister, Sheri, sustained a life-threatening brain hemorrhage on New Year's Day 2016. The miraculous doctors at Massachusetts General Hospital in Boston saved her life. Thankfully, she survived and thrived. She was not able to breathe on her own, walk, talk or eat. In her hospital bed, when she was first able to articulate some words, she said she was going to write a book. Sheri rarely ever read a book never mind writing one; especially in her condition. She was having delusions at this time so, we just said, "That is a great idea," never thinking that it would come to fruition. Sheri worked very hard in rehab and would do whatever anyone asked her to do, as she was determined to get better. With her deficits slowly improving, she started to write her story. Sheri's family is very proud of her. She has never given up and has given it all she has to get better. Her incredible hard work paid off and Sheri is doing very well and still improving.

Despite all she has been through, she has been dedicated to writing this book to raise awareness of aneurysms, brain injury, and encourage people to THINK.

- Laurie Jameson, Sheri's sister -

Introduction

Why I Wrote *Compassionate Snob*

First of all, let's get this straight, I am not a snob. Maybe I had the image of one in the past, but not anymore. The truth is, I'm now much more compassionate, hence the play on words in my title of this book. With knowledge and persistence, you can have a very comfortable life, but remember, money does not buy you happiness. It can help you acquire material things that people see. Underneath it all, we try to acquire material things to try to change the image of ourselves. Yes, image helps, but what makes you a good person is what is inside; that is our true individuality. You can have the life that you want if you don't just let things happen. YOU make them happen! Be ready to work though! Don't always judge a book by its cover. You may be surprised as to what's inside. We all tend to want to follow the crowd to be accepted. That is what I wanted, to be accepted by my professional peers, other moms, and my clients, and I thought my image would get me there … wrong again! Working on the inside is what matters. It's hard work, it takes persistence.

Baby steps and hard work will get you to your destination. "Building blocks" are the key. The unfortunate part is that some of us don't want to put in the hard work. We think it should just come to us. Life doesn't work that way. For the most part, it takes a lot of conscious hard work and determination.

With this brain bleed, a window has been opened for me, and I am very grateful for this happening. I wouldn't have paid attention otherwise! I have been violently shaken awake. Now, I have to fight for my life and I will! I have! **T H I N K**

—Sheri

• • • • | • • • •

FROM THIS MOMENT

"The only way to make sense out of change is to plunge into it, move with it, and join the dance."
—Alan Watts

"*Hello, my name is brain injury, brought to you by a bleeding stroke. You are going to be very sorry we ever met. I am going to turn your life upside down, take away your friends, turn your family against you, leave you alone and steal your identity. You will have to start all over, I will turn you into an infant who doesn't know how to chew or swallow. I will make sure you have to learn how to walk, talk, and read again. I will take the things you love to do, like reading, writing, driving, your job, your marriage, and so much away from you. You will work through months of rehab, months of pain, not being able to call or text your family because you forgot how. You will have your head shaved, horrendous headaches, and I will even steal your dreams. You may think when you leave the hospital you will be free of me, but I haven't even started yet.*

You will be completely dependent on your family. Yes, I stole all your independence along with your friends, your dignity, your ability to do the things you love to do. While I was at it I figured I might as well make sure that your family refuses to understand or educate themselves. You will be made fun of for not being able to drive, understand emotions, and much more. I will come between you and everyone you love and make you awkward and uncomfortable in public.

Had enough? Too bad, because I'm also going to make others call you lazy, accuse you of faking it, or my personal favorite, think that you're just trying to get attention. I am going to make noise unbearable, bright lights painful, make you feel like you are going crazy, and I'm even going to put thoughts and ideas in your head, and you won't know what's real or pretend. I am brain injury, and you will be sorry we ever met." (Author Unknown)

ONE OF MY good friends was getting married for the first time at fifty years old. I was very happy for her! They were having their wedding reception on New Year's Eve, 2015. I didn't really want to attend. Sorry, but it's true. Why didn't I want to go? I did not want to leave our daughter who was in her early teens. She is our only child and I am very wrapped up in her. I have a hard time leaving her. Adult interaction, festivities, parties, social gatherings are all supposed to be fun, right? Wrong. Events aren't that enjoyable for me because I worry about her; especially if I am far away. I considered this wedding to be far away for me and it was New Year's Eve. Reputably, not a good night to be on the roads.

New Year's Eve is so overrated. For the past few years, we have been quietly spending New Year's Eve at my sister's house with her family and our mutual good friends. Regardless of not wanting to go, I wanted to support my friends. I am very happy they found one another! So, I ended up choosing to go.

First of all, I had to get a dress. That was the fun part and what I really enjoyed. I had gastric sleeve surgery for weight loss only a year before and I had lost 100 pounds. I was over-weight and it was starting to impact me physically. I was tired often and it was difficult for me to stand on my feet toward the end of the day. I was a hairstylist and had to stand on my feet for long shifts, and I knew it would eventually catch up with me. Before the surgery, I ate a lot and never quite seemed full. It showed, but I tried hiding it with big stylish clothing. You see, I used to be a plus-size model. Being big was okay. I wasn't ashamed of it. Although, nothing I ever wore looked great. I was very conscientious about my looks, and I knew I could look a lot better if I were thinner and I could work more effectively. The surgery went well and I lost over 100 lbs. I felt great!

Although I was not ashamed of my weight, looks were crucial to me. I was a hairstylist for many years. All around me were current trends, fashion, and makeup. Just before the AVM rupture, I had been accepted at a Boston modeling agency for regular size older models, and I had new photos done for my portfolio. Between hairdressing and modeling, the perfect image mattered in my industry, and consequently I thought that's what life was all about.

I was excited about picking out a great dress that would be fun, stylish, and finally fit right. I found the perfect dress and it was beautiful. I rented it from "Rent-The-Runway." It is an app where you can rent designer dresses and accessories. I knew that I didn't want to wear it again. Wear the same dress twice? I don't think so! That wasn't my style, renting was the perfect option. It was easy to pick out the dress to wear. They send you two different sizes of your choice. Pick the date for delivery, and you are finished. I just had to send it back within a few days—perfect! The dresses arrived on time at my door. The first dress I tried on fit perfectly. A size 8 which I never, ever fit into. Yes, from a size 18 to a size 8. Pretty amazing. I looked great in it. Isn't that what mattered most? The dress was a black crepe, designed by Elizabeth and James. It was a Shift dress, 60s inspired, with a feathered detail on the hemline. To go with the dress, I purchased a pair of sixty-ish inspired boots. They were short, black suede, with a square high heel. Perfection!

My friend, the bride, loves the sixties. She should have been a flower-child! The dress was so perfect...Groovy, Peace and Love!

Getting ready that evening, I carefully applied my makeup. I am very good at makeup application and do it professionally. Just add a set of false eyelashes, and voila, you are good to go. My husband always comments when I have them on. There is an art to getting the right ones and applying them is easy for me, but not for everyone. So yes, I know they look good! This is where experience comes into play.

We arrived at the wedding reception. It was held in a decorated function room in the upstairs of a nice restaurant. It was only a town over from where we lived, but I still felt it was far away. The theme colors were black and red. The bride and groom looked very happy. The bride wore a lovely knee-length white dress with red cowboy boots. The groom wore a black suit with a red shirt and black tie. It was the first time I had ever met him. They were good together and looked so very happy!

We sat at a round table with some of our old friends. Coincidentally, the friends that we sat with all have one child like my husband and me. I wondered if they felt it hard to go out and leave their child, too? I knew one of them really did. We had fun eating and dancing, and of course a lot of talking naturally—isn't that what we do best?

I didn't have any drinks that evening, probably because I knew I had to drive home. It was New Year's Eve, and I wanted my husband to have a good time! Social gatherings aren't really his thing—unless it's on a golf course or at a football game. However, as usual, he was being a good sport about being there.

At midnight we took pictures. I sent some to my boss. He used to style the hair of one of my girlfriends whom I was with. So, I sent him some pictures of us at the wedding reception having fun. And of course, with the caption of "Happy New Year." We drove home happy. It was a good time. We were so glad we went and shared in the celebration.

It was a New Year—2016 now, and thankfully we got home without any incidents. Our daughter had some friends sleeping over, and we were all safe and sound! It was a good night and a safe and happy New Year!

····2····

"HOUSTON, WE HAVE A PROBLEM"

*"Identify your problems but give your power
and energy to solutions."*
—**Tony Robbins**

"CALL AN AMBULANCE!" I screamed to my husband with terror in my voice, as I started to fall. Thankfully, my husband caught me and I fell into his arms. I asked him in a weak voice losing consciousness, "Did you call the ambulance?"

That morning had started out perfectly normal. I was thankful to be home celebrating the first day of 2016 with my family, but after I ate half of a bagel, I started to feel sick. Sometimes, when I overeat, I have the potential of vomiting because of my gastric sleeve surgery, but that very rarely happens to me. I was in the bathroom off of our bedroom.

6

I remember my 16-year-old daughter coming into the bedroom knocking on the bathroom door, asking me if I was ok. I said to her as calmly as I could, "Get your father." He then casually walked into the bedroom. As I was on my way out of the bathroom, my hands started shaking up and down uncontrollably in an unusual movement! I couldn't stop them. I had no control over their movements. I vaguely remember this. I passed out leaving one eye open and one eye closed. I laid there on our bedroom floor. I probably looked good, having left my makeup on from the wedding the night before, even the false eyelashes. It really didn't matter now, did it?

Our daughter came in, and she was so scared that she slapped me really hard in the face trying to revive me. I couldn't do a thing. I vaguely remember this. My husband knew something was seriously wrong with me as I laid there unresponsive, with one eye open and one eye closed. He and my daughter probably thought it had something to do with the gastric sleeve surgery. However, I was perfectly healthy. I had all the tests! The ambulance came, and from what I hear, it took what felt to my family about ten to fifteen minutes. That's a long time when you're in crisis. My daughter was yelling at them, "Hurry, please, hurry!" I was taken out of the house in what has been described to me as a potato sack with handles. I have no recollection. The EMT's had called ahead to the local hospital so they were all ready for me. A nurse asked my husband to step into a certain room. This particular room was the same room where my husband learned that his younger and only brother had died of terminal lung cancer just three years before. My husband refused to go into that room asking, "Is my wife dead?" He wanted immediate answers.

My sister showed up at my house, after reassuring our daughter that it was just dehydration, she told her there was nothing to worry about, trying to calm her down and put her at ease. When my sister arrived at the hospital thinking that I

7

was only dehydrated, she was shocked when she saw an EMT from our town and asked him if he had brought her sister to the hospital. He told her no it was another rig, but that they had to intubate her in the ambulance. At that point, she knew something was seriously wrong!

The doctor presented the MRI results to my husband and sister. He put them up and showed them the films. They could tell even before the doctor said anything that it was critical as there was a black image the size of a tennis ball on the screen. I had a massive hemorrhage inside of my brain causing my brain to swell dangerously. The doctor said, "We aren't equipped to help her here, where do you want her to go?" "Mass General Hospital," my husband said without hesitation. He knew this was serious! My husband is usually right. They airlifted me from that hospital into Mass General Hospital (MGH) in Boston Massachusetts. They went extremely fast! Let's just say it takes about 30 - 45 minutes on a regular day to get into Boston from where I live. It only took the flight four minutes to get me there.

At Mass General Hospital, my family was thrown immediately into a situation they knew nothing about. I was unconscious and had to rely on them to make the right decisions. The seriousness of the situation came to light when the neurosurgeon resident, who looked very young, asked my family to please step into a quiet room, telling them they had to do an immediate emergency brain surgery. He made sure they understood the magnitude of the situation. I was in a very critical condition.

The first surgery performed was an emergency surgery, to stop the hemorrhage, which took around 12 hours to complete. From what I've heard, it was gruesome. They had to take a large chunk of bone out in the back of my head. They call this a "bone flap." It is sometimes replaced. However, mine didn't have to be replaced due to its location. They stopped the bleed. I survived! However, I was still in critical condition. I then developed pneumonia because I aspirated vomit, and it went into my lungs when I had first collapsed. There were also problems with my heart and blood pressure. This is when they almost lost me again. They put me on the drug that Michael Jackson died of called Propofol, while I was intubated. It was a horrifying time for my family. It was touch-and-go for a long time. My husband was very concerned that I might die. They performed several angiograms. This is where they go through your groin, up to your brain and look with a camera. I also had several tests, scans and blood work. I had one nurse assigned around the clock, just to me.

Thankfully, I recovered from the heart problem and pneumonia. As I got better, they were able to remove me from the ventilator as I was then able to breath on my own. The reason I had the brain hemorrhage was due to a congenital defect I had since birth, which I knew nothing about. It was called an AVM, arteriovenous malformation. It is a congenital defect between the arteries and veins. The blood flow from my artery put too much pressure on my vein and caused it to rupture, causing the brain hemorrhage. Now, the next step was to fix this problem. A team of specialists got together and decided how they were going to fix the AVM. They chose to put in glue plugs, so my brain would not bleed when they removed the AVM. This procedure took six hours. They did this the day before the big surgery. I had some of the best surgeons in Boston. My family was grateful, as this was a very difficult procedure. I cannot even imagine what it takes to do this extremely delicate surgery! This was again a very terrible time for my loved ones. I was dangerously close to losing it all, or becoming… well, we won't even go there!

This procedure took 8 hours. My operation was a success in their eyes! Although I had experienced a mild stroke during one of the surgeries. My eyes were now slightly out of alignment. This is why I have somewhat double vision without a prism in my glasses that I now have to wear.

I remember waking up from my induced coma, in an all-white room. From what I'm told, it was the ICU (intensive care unit). I was attached to eleven tubes. They controlled all sorts of physical things for me, such as monitoring my vitals, drugs, eating, bathroom, breathing, and brain drain. Keeping me alive was their first mission, yet at the same time, wanting desperately to leave me with some quality of life.

The trauma and medication obviously had taken a toll on my body and severely injured brain. I remember telling my nurse that I knew she was a lesbian, and how I liked them as people. She asked me how I knew that, and I replied, "Your haircut." Duh... It was a dead giveaway! At some point during this interaction, I recall she asked me "where do we go?" (meaning lesbians). Answering her question I stated, "Melissa Etheridge concerts." I stared blankly at her. I was coming out of a two-week induced coma. I was also very heavily medicated. I then heard her asking her team in the hallway at the nurse's desk if they too, thought she was gay. Yep...they all knew, and she was surprised! She told them what I had said about the haircut. I was just on A LOT of medication. All in all, I know some of this was probably a hallucination. I couldn't speak well at the time, and nobody could understand me. I never did see that nurse again. Wow, the things nurses have to put up with!

I was moved to another floor to room 818, which happens to be my birthday, by the way. This was taken by my family as a good sign. I don't know how I ended up there, or even why I was there. My ankles and wrists were tied to the bed, restraints *as* they put it in medical terms, so that I wouldn't pull my tubes and wires out. I had a shaved head with a large scar that started at the nape of my neck, then ran up and curved towards my right ear. There were huge staples holding my skin together, a feeding tube running down my esophagus, a mask and tube blowing oxygen into my mouth and nose, brain drain releasing the pressure of fluid building up inside my head, and I was hooked up to many other machines. Oh, and did I mention that I had a lot of hallucinations, that I thought were real! A couple examples of my delusions were of Oprah selling shoes to me at Nordstrom, and one of the Real Housewives was spinning around telling me how fabulous she was. Apparently, I was heavily medicated. However, I am so incredibly thankful to the staff! I never once felt physical pain that I remember. This is a miracle in itself! While being there, I just went with the flow and did what I was told, as if I were in jail. Did I think maybe they would let me out on good behavior? I was then extremely helpless and didn't have a care in the world!

My sweet nurse told me a story about her son bringing home his girlfriend for the first time. She was going to make a nice Italian dinner for all of them the weekend they visited. She made all of her Italian specialties, meatballs, sauce and chicken parmesan. After they had settled in, she asked his girlfriend if she was hungry. "We have a lot of food," she replied, offering up some of the Italian specialties that she had labored for hours to make. The girlfriend sweetly replied, "No thank you, I am a vegetarian. Do you have anything else I can eat?" I'm sure she didn't say to her what she told us! "Yeah, just go out and eat the grass!" We laughed and laughed. It was so funny! Cooking for all that time, never mind shopping, and come to find out she's a vegetarian! How does your son forget to tell you that? My nurse was funny and kind. I will always remember her telling us that story. We all needed a good laugh!

I'm sure being a nurse is a very depressing and stressful job. I have since found a new respect for anyone that is in this profession. You have to be an extraordinary person and be very good at what you do. Luckily, my nurse was and so was her assistant.

In the beginning, I was not allowed to eat "real food." The staff and my family were told not to give me any, probably because I had a choking issue. I didn't like the feeding tube at all. I kept trying to pull it out of my nose. I had been successful at this and proud as a peacock when I succeeded. Putting it back in, now that's a different story. After pulling it out for the third time, they did a swallowing test and my doctor finally said to feed me some pancakes. It was the first real solid food I had eaten in weeks! I can only imagine since I don't remember it. However, I do love pancakes now.

After a few weeks, the day came when they sat me in a chair next to my bed. They used a patient lift to raise me while secured in a sling with the lift facilitating the move. I remember I didn't last long sitting in a chair, maybe only ten minutes. I was very dizzy, and I didn't feel so good. I also remember that they gave me a swallowing test, which I passed. So off I went to Spaulding Rehab Hospital by ambulance.

·····3·····

BROKEN DOLL

BROKEN GIRLS BLOSSOM INTO WARRIORS

AT SPAULDING REHABILITATION Hospital, the room was nice, but I honestly didn't know where I was. To my left was a large window that looked over the streets of Boston. To my right was a whiteboard hanging on the wall. This was where my schedule for the day was written out for me. Boy, did this whiteboard keep me very busy! I wanted to rest, but they explained to me how important it was to my recovery for me to keep moving. I tried to relax and take it easy. I thought that was recovering. Boy, was I wrong!

I was determined to get better and was faithfully sticking to my schedule dictated by the whiteboard. Physical therapy was up first. So, the first thing was to get dressed, with help of course. This was when reality hit me. I couldn't walk! Did I mention this? Yes, one of the worst things that affected me was not being able to walk anymore, something I took for granted! My equilibrium was completely off and I felt like I had no control over my legs. The therapists would sit me up, and I would fall over unless they were holding on to me. I also was no longer able to talk correctly, and my fine motor skills were affected, especially in my right hand. I couldn't hold a pen and a lot of my everyday body movements were now extremely difficult.

So off I went in a wheelchair, with my physical therapist for an hour. The therapy room had beautiful glass windows from floor to ceiling, bright and cheery as it could be. I performed all sorts of different types of exercises that they prescribed for me. Then I went to group therapy. Here, 8-10 patients sat around tables put together in a large square. We played a different game every day. (Didn't anyone get the memo about how I hate playing games?) It was therapeutic of course. The games that were played used hand-eye coordination, and memory. We also had to answer questions about daily events. So, I tried to watch the news with my breakfast every morning. During Speech Therapy, I sat in a room sometimes in my hospital bed, doing all sorts of workbook activities. I was assigned a Speech Therapist that did many things with me. I participated wholeheartedly in everything I did.

It seemed that so many people were worse off than me, hurting in all kinds of ways. I saw many unfortunate things that I couldn't even imagine! I remember one time, as I was being wheeled down the hall in my trusty wheelchair, there was a man being escorted down the hall by 5 or 6 nurses. They were helping him walk with braces on his arms and legs, hooked up to all kinds of machinery. Yes, I was fortunate! After seeing what he had to go through, this gave me such compassion for him and made me realize how thankful and lucky I was.

However, there were many times that I would get discouraged, especially when I looked in the mirror. I saw my bald head with a deep scar that I couldn't see that well; but I knew it was there. I still tried to make the best of things. My incision had the appearance of an elephant trunk. With the hallucinations, I had thought that the many staples that were implanted in my shaved head were pink rhinestones! I guess this proves that the drugs were good. I would ask everyone that I saw (if I had enough energy to), "Do you want to see my elephant?"

Outside of my room usually stood a couple of nurses. Every night, I remember asking them to give me a particular drug. I forget now what it was called, but it helped me sleep. I could hear people screaming at night, yes I needed those drugs. Every day I got a shot of something in my stomach, I believe it was a blood thinner.

I let them do what they had to do. It was their job, and I wasn't going to make it harder than it already was. Being negative only results in an adverse outcome. I tried to think of others. Giving a shot must be an awful thing to have to do. Just as much as giving someone an eyebrow wax is no fun either. Being a good patient isn't easy. I kept thinking, "I will try my best to make it easy for you to do your job."

My family was very supportive. My husband, daughter, and sister were exceptional! My parents came as much as they could (they are getting older). The trip into town was very hard on them, let alone seeing their daughter in such an awful state. Their lives had been turned upside down. This tragedy didn't just happen to me. It happened to my whole family.

I loved visitors and was so thankful that some of my best friends came in to see me. I still really couldn't grasp the situation yet, but I understood some of it. The gummy bears that one of my close friends brought me was such a treat! CANDY? I felt like I was Elf with the syrup! And I ate them all! I was so delighted that some of my good friends came to visit me! The next day I woke up with the worst stomach ache of my life. They wanted me to go to physical therapy. I tried to go, but I couldn't do it. My stomach hurt too bad. I didn't feel right. A nurse came in and gave me a suppository. Seriously? Now I wish I had the strength to yell at the nurse and tell her that I had never been so mistreated. I wanted to get her fired for only doing her job. It was humiliating! It wasn't her fault that I chose to eat all the candy. When I asked to be brought into the bathroom, I was in for an even bigger surprise. A nurse had to stay and watch me. As if the suppository wasn't embarrassing enough, now this? No, this isn't happening! As I sat writhing in pain, this just topped it off! I had now hit an all-time low.

Oh, and if that wasn't bad enough, I found out they had a nickname for me too! There was a shower next to me in the bathroom so I would grab the shower curtain and hide behind it while I went. They had to stay there with me to make sure that I didn't fall. Oh, my new nickname, you ask? It was, "The Wizard," (referencing Dorothy in the Wizard of Oz, asking "who's behind the curtain?") Who made that one up? So, let's move on with it! I missed almost a week of physical therapy due to this candy eating issue. I thought it was only a day! That tells you how potent the drugs were.

·····4·····

CRACKED EGG

"She was a girl who knew how to be happy even when she was sad, and that's important."
—**Marilyn Monroe**

EVEN THOUGH MY insides came out emotionally, over-all I had learned a lot. I was happy to be leaving Spaulding Rehabilitation Hospital. A man loaded me into a wheelchair van, as the wind blew off the water. It was cold, so I was dressed warmly. I was on my way to stay at a nursing home/ rehab facility (It was a nursing home. I don't care what they say). My sister worked there, and I was much closer to my family being a patient there. I was pleased about this and very excited to be going. Who would've ever thought that I would be happy going to a nursing home?

The ride, however, was not fun. The driver had two different radios going. One was rap music and the other was constant chatter on the transport radio. It was also very bright out. I wished they had taken me to the bathroom before I left as my bladder felt like it was going to explode. I didn't feel well when I arrived. Now I know why. The brain injury had caused this feeling. The light, the noise, and the motion caused me to get nauseated. Here's a tip...wear sunglasses! I wasn't aware of any of this until later. It is very apparent to me now! People that have been affected by brain trauma are usually very sensitive to weather, light, movement and noises. Nobody ever told me this.

My sister worked at this nursing home as a social worker. Thankfully, I had my own room. It was a lovely place, as far as nursing homes go. This facility was nice and it didn't smell like urine. The greatest thing was, I didn't have to do group therapy anymore; although I did still have to do physical therapy, occupational therapy, and speech therapy.

The nurses were excellent at my new residence. Like I stated before, I like nurses. I have great respect for them. What they do for other people is a Godsend.

When I arrived in my room, some of the staff came into my room to welcome me. I think they may have expected someone like my sister. Well, what they got is the opposite of her...me! My sister is so soft-spoken, compassionate, sweet and keeps her opinions to herself. She should wear a halo! I'm very serious. Also, I have a different fashion sense and more creative, and she's not so much. although, she is the angel on earth and I'm not. I'm not as soft-spoken and much more opinionated. I just won't let people walk all over me. Not that my sister does either, but we go about it in different ways. I'm just more direct. I do not sugar-coat things. I tell it like it is. I have come to learn that some people don't like this. Some people don't like to hear the truth! Well, my truth anyway. Believe me, I don't try to say things in a mean way. That's okay though; I make life way more interesting! Maybe that's why my daughter says I can be dramatic sometimes...I am not a drama queen. I'm not a queen at all! Well, maybe sometimes a princess. Everybody has an opinion. Even if you don't agree you should still give them respect and listen to their perceptions.

When the nurse came in to give me my pills, I took them in applesauce. I assume they did it this way because they go down easier. I was given my medication morning, noon, and night. Oh, and my blood pressure was taken morning, noon, and night and whether I was standing up, sitting down or laying down.

Every time someone used the call buzzer next to their bed to call for a nurse, I heard it. It was right outside my door. At the nursing home, they all wake up early. So needless to say, I woke early too. Don't they know that brain injury patients require a lot of sleep? We do! This is when your brain heals and repairs itself. Buzz, buzz! Nurses waking me up to take my blood pressure, or even worse − to have my blood drawn, or administering medications, were exhausting. No wonder I sometimes hid underneath the covers! I just wanted to be left alone with my Dunkin' Donuts iced decaf coffee. Heaven-sent beverage that I looked forward to receiving each morning that my sister worked. She's such an angel.

I am blessed with many angels and I thank God for my husband, daughter, sister, and the rest of my family that helped me. I appreciated it, although I had a hard time showing it. Being independent and then having to rely on others was very, very hard for me to do. My husband and daughter were amazing. They came and visited me all the time! They washed my clothes, brought me food, they even brought in the dog! Every night they changed me into my pajamas and made sure I was comfortable. I'm sure there was nothing but discomfort for them. They even brought in a blanket that one of my clients had crocheted for us for our anniversary. We had nicknamed it "The Dead Body blanket," because it was very heavy and felt like dead weight on you when you were covered with it. Did you know that heavy blankets are good for anxiety? That's what a nurse told me.

"Rise and shine. It's time for your shower" I was awakened by an aide saying this to me. Is she serious? I asked myself. I didn't know what time it was, but it was very early. I was the first shower of the day, and all I remember was that it was cold as …! An aide wheeled me into the shower and helped me. She actually taught me how to wash.

I had to learn how to do many things all over again, and showering was just one of them. It wasn't easy not being able to walk or talk correctly. I told people a lot that I sounded like Matthew McConaughey (an American actor who is southern). It was especially hard not having any fine motor skills in my right hand. I was a righty before all of this happened. Think of me as a baby. I could not walk, dress or bathe myself. People had a very difficult time understanding me as I spoke like a two year old child, and I even had to wear a brief as I had some incontinence. I had to relearn everything. I wore a gait belt which was wrapped around my torso like a harness, so someone could catch me if I fell. My therapist came to my room to get me daily. I was wheeled down to the rehab room. I spent a lot of time there, over 3 hours every day.

As days went on, I started to get anxious about getting out of there and going home. I wanted by own environment and some normalcy. One day a nurse's aide brought me my lunch. She set the tray down in front of me. I lifted the plastic cover only to find a whole plate of Brussel sprouts. Setting the cover back on my lunch, I looked at the aid and politely said that "this isn't my lunch". She told me it was mine. Nope, then I looked again as if they had disappeared. No, they had not! I repeated my statement and slid my plate full of Brussel sprouts toward her. They kindly brought me another lunch.

I hated the weekends when everyone got to go home. On the weekends the staff changed. My physical therapist was different too. I really didn't like it. That's where I wanted to be…HOME, you know Home Sweet Home? I know I had to learn to try and make the best of it. I kept thinking, if you're well-behaved in prison, don't you get released earlier for good behavior? Well, why couldn't I go home? They weren't having it, believe me, I tried.

My blood pressure was very low, so I was wrapped up in a stomach binder, and my legs were wrapped up in gauze to right above my knees. I also had to sleep at a 30-degree angle. Never mind that at one point, everybody had to wear a face mask because my white blood count was low. They did not want me to get an infection. There were even masks left outside my door for everyone that came in contact with me!

"Today we're going to try a walker," said my physical therapist. I was always up for anything. I would get better. I just had to! She taught me how to use a walker. I would carefully walk with my trusty walker back to my room, holding on for dear life! I was always looking down towards my feet. I realize now it was due to the light and motion, all the stimulation that we take for granted. Moving my neck was very difficult at that time, also the pattern of the hall rug made me feel sick – not that I didn't like the look of the rug. It just didn't like me. It gave me the feeling similar to motion sickness. But, I fought it - it was me against the rug!

Although I was making strides daily, I had such a long way to go. My appearance had changed so much. I had lost twenty-six more pounds during this time and my head was completely shaven. During physical therapy one day, an older woman said something about "that boy over there" and pointed to me. She thought I was a boy? Now I know there's a problem; but she was right. I did look like a boy! I had a shaved head, was very thin and lanky, wearing a t-shirt and a pair of sweatpants, and had no makeup on! I lived for that stuff! But not anymore, makeup and hair were the last things on my agenda. Ahh! Hearing someone that speaks their truth was very refreshing. Even though she was a hundred and one (yes, I'm serious)! She ended up becoming a friend of mine. I was very sad when I later found out about her passing. I had visited her once after I left. I would've gone and visited more if only I could have.

One day my speech therapist came to my room to work with me. She normally would have me write and color. But today, she asked me to sing! "Oh, come on and sing!" Seriously? Weren't these stupid tests and coloring in coloring books enough? Now you want me to sing? "NO, I won't do it!", I said stubbornly. She was adamant. I only did it just to get rid of her. She asked me to sing the first song that I remembered from being little. So, I somewhat sang *Delta Dawn*. I remembered the words! Somehow it even surprised me. Knowing the words to that song brought on unexpected tears. That song brought me back into my father's station wagon, putting in an eight-track tape, and singing every word! I sang that song back then over and over again. "Delta Dawn, what's that flower you have on? Could it be a painted rose from days gone by?" And yes, I could remember every word. "I remembered!" I cried after having such a powerful memory. My speech therapist probably didn't expect that. Neither did I. I guess, the music evokes a lot of memories, and it speaks to you.

Now that this AVM rupture has happened to me, I listen to music a lot. It is my friend. I listen to the words of songs much more carefully now. I try to put myself in the songwriter's place to understand them better. I now use music and songs to express myself.

••••• 5 •••••

GOODBYE GIRL

Find the good in goodbye

IT HAD BEEN over three months since the night of my injury. So you can imagine that I was all ready to go home when my husband came to pick me up at the nursing home. They had already done the home evaluation. They had to remove some of the scatter rugs and put a bar up in the shower, so that I wouldn't slip or fall. There were places in the house that were entirely off limits. I had become a rule abider because all I ever wanted was to go home. So, I was packed and ready to go!

While driving home towards my house, everything looked familiar. I had been warned that I should wear sunglasses on the ride home. It helps with the motion sickness. Now they tell me! So, I did. We stopped and went through the Dunkin Donuts drive-thru for an iced decaf coffee. My favorite! I love them! I think I'm addicted! As we turned down our street, I started to cry. It was out of sheer joy. A smiley face balloon was placed on our mailbox by a friendly neighbor. It meant so much! It felt exhilarating to be home finally!

I took it slow, going from my walker to my wheelchair. Getting acclimated to my old surroundings, which felt new again, was a surreal moment for me. During the home inspection, my physical therapist at the nursing home had put down orange duct tape everywhere so that I would be reminded to slow down. I had duct tape on the sink in the kitchen, the sharp edges of the coffee tables, bathroom, etc.... I could only get into the bathroom with my walker because the wheelchair didn't fit. So, a commode was placed next to my bed, that way everyone in my family felt more secure and they could sleep better knowing I was safe if I got up on my own. Yes, things were different. VERY different!

One night shortly after I had first arrived at home, we were sitting down as a family at the dinner table and I made the comment that I wished I was dead. I was told to never say that again – and I haven't. At this time, I didn't have the mental capacity to know that this was very hurtful to my family. If I had the mental capacity at the time, I would have put it much differently. This was my way of saying that I hated the situation we had all been put in. But without a filter I would say out loud whatever came across my mind. Like a child, I did not know any better. It was like telling someone they're fat or ugly. I once told a family member that I was going to make her a candle, as she loved Yankee Candles. She then replied, "What is it going to smell like?" I replied "Pee, one that smells like pee". Since I had to sleep with a commode next to my bed at night, all I could smell was pee. So, that is what came to my mind and out of my mouth.

I was a walking, talking brat, without a filter. I frequently was told this by my mother. She would say to me, "Put your filter on, Sheri" in a voice that irritated me. That only agitated me more. I finally snapped at her one day. "Did I ever have one to begin with?" I said sharply! I was always a direct person, but now I was sometimes mean when I said some things. At that time, I didn't care, it was my truth. I felt nobody wanted to listen to my comments and my opinions no longer mattered.

As weeks went by and I began to slowly heal, I would go out for rides with family and friends. When I would go out somewhere, the only noticeable thing I had to others was a shaved head with a prominent scar and a walker. Nobody knew what was wrong with me. I felt I still looked the same. Yes, I had been through hell and back. But, I was still the same person and becoming somewhat different but in a better way! Humbled, I guess you would call it.

Our daughter is the most important person in my life! She was my job even though it never felt like a job to me. Although my husband and I raise her together in our home, she and I were inseparable. We had never spent a night apart until that dreadful day of my injury when I was hospitalized. Then we were separated for months, three to be exact, but who was counting? I often think how horrific that must have been for her. My family told me, when I first woke up and was barely conscious, I mumbled "how is my daughter"? It is an innate feeling in us always to have our children as our primary concern, not ourselves.

She was a teenager, and at that age they are so busy creating their own lives, wanting to be independent. Most parents know how that goes. I wanted her to spread her wings and fly, even if it's hard for me. What matters is her living her best life. It is bittersweet.

Imagine having children and not being able to raise them the way you had intended. My husband fortunately, took over this role. I am very proud of what he has accomplished! We are different in our approach to child-raising. Believe it or not, I'm more of a pushover and he is more of the disciplinarian. He's of the mind that a child needs to learn through teachings of the cruel hard world. There were a lot of things I was no longer able to do for my daughter. For example, I could not teach her to drive or help her get her license. My husband took her to pick out her prom dresses and had to help with all of the college preparation. I was very happy that he was able to do this for all of us, but as a mother I wish I could have done this for her. These tasks were always my job and I loved everyone them.

I was forced to make the separation from her, cold turkey. Most mothers know that the separation is coming and slowly morph into that transitional phase by taking their child to get their driver's license, going on college tours, being involved in schooling and extracurricular activities. I very much wanted to share in those experiences and I couldn't do any of it.

The year of my brain injury was also second half of our daughter's junior year in high school. She looked beautiful all dressed up for her junior prom. I was so proud of her. We went to see her have pictures taken at a local park with all of her classmates. It was my first outing that included the local parents. Although I knew this day was about the kids, I felt almost invisible to most of the women I used to know and associate with. They looked at me as if I had risen from the dead. I was lucky if I got a hello. It was a life transforming experience for me. Everything seemed different to me now. It was as though I was looking at the players and the situation through a different lens and seeing the truth. The school stuff had all become a competition. Now, I see it ever so clearly from a spectator's point of view. The mothers seemed so concerned if their daughter had the best dress, the best hair, and the best makeup. I thought 'my God, that used to be me!"

The reality of it was that I was grateful just to make my daughter's bed by noon! Topping it off with her blanket that she has had since she was a baby and a stuffed bear she had won with writing on its belly that says, "I love you", took every ounce of physical effort for me to do. Some days it took me 20 minutes to make that bed; but I was determined to do it for her. This small gesture made me feel like I was still her mother and I was still taking care of her. Being a mother there are things that we do daily that go unnoticed. We just do them effortlessly because they are our children and we want the best for them. My daughter is and will always be the most important person in my life. I heard this saying a long time ago and it will always be true. "It's like your heart has legs and is walking around."

My husband and daughter were on their own now and I could not do a thing about it. They were more concerned about me and my condition. With the exception of making the beds and doing small chores around the house, my main job was getting better. If I didn't take care of myself who would take care of them? That was my job now. Getting better was my first priority.

A week or so after I returned home from the rehab/nursing home, my daughter gave me a stack of get-well cards and there were a lot! My husband and daughter had been so busy with everything they had to endure, that they had forgotten about the cards I had received from many well-wishers. Our lives had changed so suddenly and drastically in a split second. We had been shaken to the core by an unexpected force. So this gesture from our daughter and friends had meant so much. You will never know. Unbeknownst to anyone, our daughter had collected and saved every one of them and tucked them away in her room, keeping them for me. I couldn't believe it! All that time she had been saving them. This was a beautiful gesture that I will never forget. It is hard for me to express how very touching this act of kindness was to me. I still have them today. Just thinking of the people that wished me well, knowing I will never see some of them again, makes me choke up. As I was a hairstylist for over 30 years, most of them were from my clients. They meant a lot to me, and since I left so suddenly, I never got the chance to say goodbye.

····6····

PUTTING THE PIECES BACK DIFFERENTLY

"You never know how strong you are,
until being strong is your only choice."
—Bob Marley

HELL WAS STARTING, and I didn't even know it. As the old saying goes: *"Be careful what you wish for; you just might get it."* Yes, I was home, but I couldn't walk without the aid of my walker or get around without my trusty wheelchair. I had a lot to do now that I was home. I would do what I was told. I knew that rules were put in place for a reason. The rules that they gave to me were so I didn't get hurt. My acceptance of the rules made my family much more comfortable knowing that I would be somewhat safe in their absence.

I also realized that I was very slow at everything. There were many things I couldn't do because of the hemorrhagic stroke. Like I said before, in my right hand, my fine motor skills were gone. That means that I have a hard time writing and doing the simplest of chores. My speech sounded Southern, and my eyesight was off. I had slight double vision. But the worst of all was a feeling that I was left with inside my head… a vertigo feeling. There was this continuous pressure sensation. It felt kind of like walking around with a cinderblock on my head…. It's so tough to describe, and yes, I constantly have this feeling. My neurosurgeon said it would be one of the last things to go away. I can only hope that he's right. What I have come to learn is that it takes a very long time for the brain to heal. A lot longer than anyone would imagine. I thought I would be better in a few months. No, I was very wrong it can often take years. I had been provided with some help at home. I had a visiting nurse, a physical therapist, occupational therapist, and a speech therapist. I had very low blood pressure for quite a while, so the visiting nurse and my sister would keep track of it in a notebook. I had a calendar that I lived by to keep track of my medical appointments. Believe me, there were a lot! Everyone would write in it when they could come by and help or visit so I could keep track of my daily schedule.

My family was taking care of me when the visiting staff weren't there. I really thought I could do it all on my own but ended up struggling quite often. I tried so hard not to show it. I am sure it must have been tough for them to watch. Along with filling my weekly pill box of prescribed medication, my family had to take care of me continuously. This is where you have to trust others, I am very thankful that I can trust my family.

Before I had the brain surgery, I did everything myself. I didn't think anyone was listening to me. I used to be louder and in control. It took a lot of energy for me to talk now. I spoke softly because of this. I was physically weak and every-thing required much more effort. The little things that we take for granted every day were now a huge challenge for me. I kept motivated by thinking, I will prove to my family that I can and will recover! I kept this to myself. I did all of the exercises that I was given...morning, noon, and night. I was determined to get better. My physical therapist also told me that I was going to learn to walk without a walker. This made me extremely nervous because she made it seem like it was no big deal. It was to me! "Can't you see, I can't walk without a walker?" I loudly said, so frustrated with what I felt was a delay in my progress. Slowly but surely, I was relearning to walk and talk again. Do you know what the worst of all this was? It was having my independence taken away. Not being able to drive and having to depend on everybody for everything, even something as simple as my favorite morning iced coffee.

At first my schedule was packed with visitors and helpers, but then I slowly noticed that people weren't coming around that much anymore. The initial drama was over, however, not for my family or me. The problem is that on the outside, I was starting to look like myself, so that made most people feel better. However, for some of my closest friends, seeing me was difficult. As I have been told, it was tough for them to see me like this, so this is why some people chose not to visit. It's easier for them I guess. I also stayed away to lessen their pain. I wasn't that easy to deal with either, which didn't help any.

My emotions were all over the place. I would laugh, cry, and get easily agitated. I had no filter at that time, I said whatever came to my mind. For example, when I was at the doctor's office, I would ask people why they were there; or I would tell someone that I didn't like them. I would say any-thing to anyone. No wonder people didn't come to visit me. They didn't want to be told what I really thought! Now that I know better, I keep that type of thing to myself. My brain had to heal. Everyone is different and so is every brain injury.

I cut a lot of people out. I wanted to get smarter and learn new things, and unfortunately, this included new people. I had no use for things I already knew so I pushed some people away. Looking back now, I wish I hadn't been so forceful in doing that, and I wished my friends had understood more about what can happen to a person with a brain injury. I acted that way when I first came home because my brain still had a lot of healing to do.

One day, I went into Mass General Hospital to see my neurosurgeon that had performed my emergency surgery, Dr. William E. Butler, MD. I wanted to thank him. Thank God, he was on call that fateful day, along with the team that helped him! I guess you can't have much fun on New Year's Eve knowing that you have to be "on" the next day doing neurosurgery. It makes you profoundly aware that it takes an incredibly-skilled team to perform this kind of work. I am extremely grateful for what they did for me. If it weren't for all of their knowledge, skills and perseverance I would not be functioning at this level, if at all. All the learning I have done about the intricacies of the brain, I can't even begin to imagine. Holding someone's life in their hands must be an amazing responsibility. My husband told me there was a sign framed on his wall that listed the top 100 brain surgeons in the world and he was one of the top ten! I remember doing exercises in his waiting room and holding on to my walker. Going into his office he asked my husband and sister why I wasn't walking yet. I felt for a moment he didn't realize all the hard work I was doing to get to where I was. I really had no questions for him. Except, when was I going to get better? He told me I would get better, but it will take a lot of hard work, and it would be a very slow process. At this time, I was unaware that by slow he meant years! They really don't know. Every brain injury is different. I gave him a thank you card with a glittery heart on the front. What do you say to a man that saved your life? Thank you somehow just wasn't good enough. I had also told him that I would write a book. I gave him a hug and I was off. Little did he know, that when I left his office. I realized what I really want to do is give back. I couldn't articulate my feelings back then. I never really have been challenged like this before, until after my brain hemorrhage, and I rose to the occasion. I am a very positive, determined person now.

I remember another time when my mother took me to my first appointment with my primary care physician after having the hemorrhage. She had to drive me because I was unable to drive. When you have a brain injury like mine, they take your license away and make you take a special test after a year. I went to see my primary doctor quite regularly, so I was comfortable there. I didn't want my parents to treat me any differently. I just wanted them to enjoy their lives in retirement. They were both retired and remarried. Live your life and enjoy it!

But, I needed assistance and maneuvering was tricky, especially in unfamiliar areas. My primary care doctor came in. It had been a while since I had seen him. I didn't have any questions. I just needed to be seen by him because I was now back home. Well, of course, my mother had questions! So, she seriously asked my doctor, "What should we do about Sheri's dandruff?" With all of my serious health problems, this is what she asked? You have got to be kidding me? Like I didn't know what to do? Shutting my eyes, I thought to myself, please just take me home. I still cannot believe she asked that question! My whole life is upside down and she's asking about my dandruff?! (Did I tell you that my profession was a hairstylist?)

As we pulled into my driveway, she went ahead of me to unlock the door. Suddenly I heard a voice ask, "Are you all right?" I looked around and grabbed my phone to see if the voice was coming from it. Realizing that it wasn't coming from my phone, I heard the voice ask again, "Are you all right?"

As I was looking all around the car, I replied, "Yes, what do you think, of course, I'm fine." I messed with the buttons on the car radio thinking that the car was talking to me through "On-Star" or something. My mother was at the car window signaling me to roll it down. I rolled it down asking her (I was annoyed now) "What is wrong with your car? Where is that voice coming from?" She pointed to my neck saying, "I think it's your Life Alert." "Oh that," I sheepishly replied. It was tucked under my turtleneck. I had forgotten that I even had it on. I pulled it out from under my shirt saying, "Sorry, I must have hit the button by mistake." So now you know how I was kept safe. I wore a gait belt and a Life Alert. So, if I fell they could find me and pick me up I could just press a button for help. I was officially a contender for the "I've fallen and can't get up" commercial. Isn't that comforting?

On top of all of this I had some heart issues. So, in I went to see the cardiologist. Now remember, my perceptions were off and my social filter was gone. Everyone in the waiting room was watching me when we were leaving, or so I thought. So, I turned around and stuck my tongue out at the entire waiting room audience! At least now they had something to look at! Really...how rude, I thought. I didn't realize that I was only headed to get my blood tested 3 times in 20-minute intervals and I had to return to that same room. While we were sitting there waiting, I had told my husband what I had done. He said, "No wonder why they were looking at me with looks that could kill." Together we just burst out laughing. It was a great moment. It felt so good because believe me, there hadn't been many laughs in a very long time.

I also went to Braintree Rehab. I was excited to go and meet new people. Everyone there had something wrong and of course were concerned with their own illness. I talked to everyone. I guess it's the hairstylist in me. I made conversations with people I didn't know. That's right. I knew how to talk to people. Although talking was difficult for me physically. I wasn't intimidated. I had experience talking with all sorts of people while doing their hair. That was part of my job, which I desperately missed. I never thought I would say that. Never say never!

At Braintree Rehab, they really did try to help me. I was, however, drowning in co-pays…twenty dollars for each discipline. I went to three disciplines two times a week for months. Sadly, my life was turning into a pile of bills and medication. "Don't worry about it," my husband said. He reassured me and said everything was going to be fine. My husband was so very patient with me. I was a walking, talking, honest brat! And he loved me through it all. "Put your filter on," was told to me quite often. I slowly learned that, so now I know what to say out loud and what to keep to myself.

After many months of rehab, I was finally able to walk without my walker. It was so freeing and empowering to know I overcame such a huge obstacle, although I always had it close by, just in case. One day, one of my therapists had me walk the halls all by myself. She picked up a magazine and said walk and read this aloud. I couldn't do it. She then asked me why. "I can't read Spanish," I replied. Yes, the magazine was written in Spanish. We both cracked up!

Before my AVM rupture - September 2015

A picture from my modeling portfolio taken three months
before the AVM rupture.

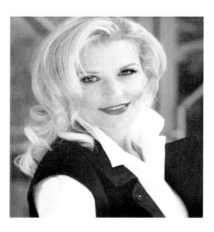

New Year's Eve 2016 - the night before the AVM struck.

Celebrating the wedding of a close friend on New Year's Eve.
11 hours later my life changed forever.

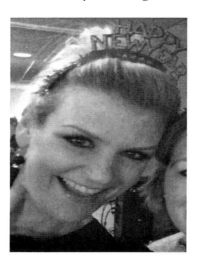

Post-AVM rupture - January 2016

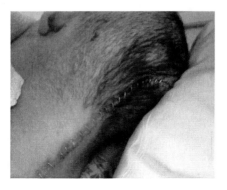

After the AVM ruptured, I had 16 hours of emergency craniotomy surgery. With another 2 surgeries to follow lasting 9 and 18 hours respectively. These are the staples that were in my head. Part of my bone in my skull was removed. I now have a significant dent in the back of my head.

Post-AVM rupture January 2016

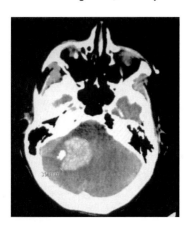

An x-ray of my brain hemorrhage. It was 39 mm in size, which is equivalent to the size of the face on a man's watch.

Post-surgery – January 2016

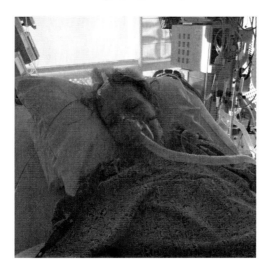

This is me after a 12-hour emergency surgery was performed. I was then put into a medically induced coma for about a week. I have no recollection of this.

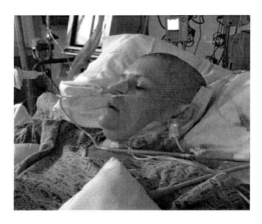

Some point at Massachusetts General Hospital. This picture was taken to show our daughter what to expect before she came to visit me for the first time.

February 2016

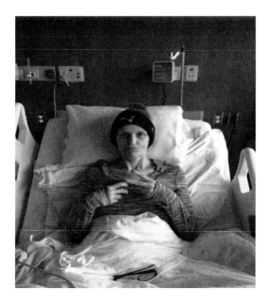

After coming out of the coma and my brain swelling went down, I was transported to Spaulding Rehabilitation Hospital in Cambridge.

At Spaulding Rehabilitation Hospital – February 2016

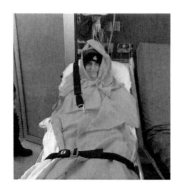 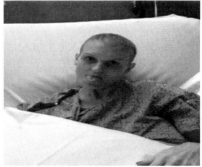

Still a Brat, but now I had no filter. NONE!

April 2016

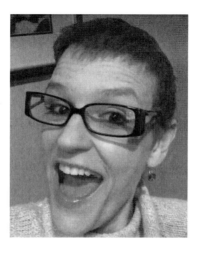

Finally, home and my hair is growing back. Needless to say, this was the least of my problems. No hair, don't care! I had a lot of other things to work on!

One year after coming home - 2017

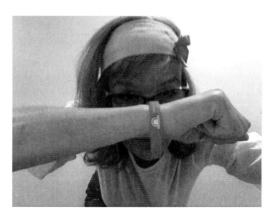

I read something about how nobody knows about our condition. It's not like we wear a cast or anything? So, I wrapped an ace bandage around my head and stuck my survivor's pin in it to try to get our point across! This is when I became a part of the Brain Aneurysm Foundation.

August 2016

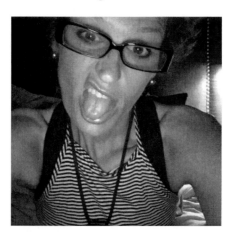

One of the only pictures I have wearing my life alert necklace!

September 2017

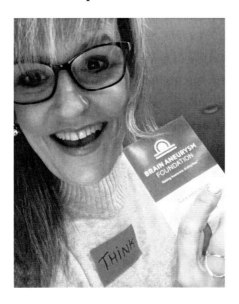

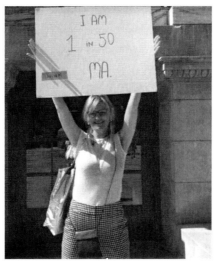

I finally found the Brain Aneurysm Foundation!
My first time at the state house in Boston advocating with the Brain Aneurysm Foundation!
September is declared brain Aneurysm Month.

April 2017 – Fenway Park Brain Aneurysm Foundation Annual Race

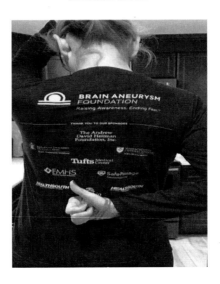

This is the t-shirt everyone received that participated in Brain Aneurysm Foundation Annual Walk for Awareness held at Fenway Park in Boston. There are so many people that have been touched by this awful disease. So many that care and do as much as they can to raise awareness! Together we are making a difference and knowledge is power!

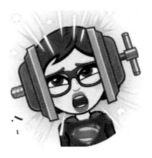

I now use this image from the Bitmoji app often. It explains how I feel every day inside my head. I chose the uniform because I identify with Super Girl. I might have some sort of superpower! (Just kidding!)

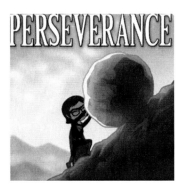

Dealing with this injury has been like climbing up a mountain and I'm fighting like hell! I even surprise myself! YOU CAN TOO!

August 2018

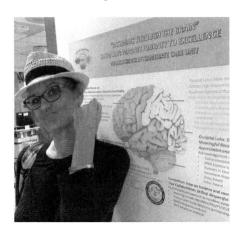

TOGETHER WE CAN FIGHT THIS!
#AWARENESSMATTERS ❤

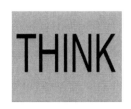

····· 7 ·····

THINK...

"Do not dwell in the past, do not dream of the future, concentrate the mind on the Present moment."
—Buddha

WHY IS THE word "THINK" so important to me? Well, when I came out of the Propofol induced coma, that I was kept in for over a week to reduce the swelling, I kept on saying that a lot of kids today don't think. What I meant was, that many kids and even adults don't choose to use their own brains. I personally think it is due to society being addicted to technology. Our brain is our own personal computer. Our children have the world at their fingertips, but we foolishly give in to providing them with the most up-to date technology because we don't want them to be left out. Unfortunately, we all seem to be getting addicted to technology and we are not using our brains as much anymore. I won't get into much here; but you get the point.

44

One day, I had a great idea! Well, I thought it was. When the physical therapist had visited my house and did a home evaluation, she had put down bright orange duct tape in places around my home. The tape signified where I was to slow down (caution tape). My idea was, I could buy orange duct tape and write the word "THINK" on the tape. I would then give it to people as a nice gesture. I had nothing to physically give them, not that anyone expected anything in return. I just wanted them to have something from me. So, a piece of orange duct tape it was, with a word written on it that said, "THINK". Yes, that was my gift. It was a message to people to SLOW DOWN and THINK! I made it into bookmarks, put it on cell phones and on computers. I thought of it as a kind gesture that was given to people who had done nice things for me. An orange piece of duct tape was all that I physically had to give them, and of course, my friendship.

People don't always realize that it is hard for me to write. I couldn't write well. As I am writing this, I am using my left hand. Even though this has been a huge challenge, it has made my brain stronger. I have had to relearn and retrain my brain. I now write with my left hand due to the lack of my fine motor skills in my right hand.

Please use your brain in this fast-paced world. It is a miraculous organ and it is sadly taken for granted until you lose its complete and complex ability Think of it as your own personal computer! People don't think a lot for themselves today. As it has been told to me quite often, if you don't use it, you will lose it. We take most things for granted. "SLOW DOWN and THINK!"

••••• 8 •••••

UNFILTERED

"You're going to come across people in your life who will say all the right words at all the right times. But in the end, it's always their actions you should judge them by. It's actions not words that matter."
—Nicholas Sparks

WE WERE TOLD that aneurysms are often hereditary, so my mother was tested for aneurysms because of my situation. The test is an MRA (a colored MRI) and it revealed two aneurysms in her brain. They are measured and if an aneurysm has the potential to rupture, they may choose to operate. One of her aneurysms had to be operated on because of its size; it had the potential to rupture. Her second aneurysm was small and would need to be monitored. There are three different tests in doing this: computed topography, magnetic resonance imaging, and angiography. These tests determine the size of an aneurysm.

One day after my mother had recently returned home from this surgery, and my sister had to run a quick errand for her. My sister had taken me with her to a local grocery store. It was good for me to go for a ride. The stimulation of the car ride was good for me with everything whizzing by. Oh, the things we take for granted! We pulled into the grocery store parking lot, and my sister parked her small SUV. Upon leaving she told me not to go anywhere. Like I was planning on that, I could hardly walk. Really? Seriously? Whatever!

Come to THINK about it, I guess she knew me! Alone in the car, I looked out the window to see a smaller version of a grocery cart. PERFECT! I thought to myself! I got out of her car without my walker holding on to her car for dear life. Somehow, I managed to pick up the shopping cart and put it in the back of her SUV! I was determined. I picked it up all by myself. I was so proud that I somehow had managed to get it into the back of her car seemingly unnoticed! Sitting back down in the front passenger seat satisfied and proud, I crossed my legs as I quietly laughed to myself! As we were leaving the parking lot, she saw me laughing and wanted to know what was so funny. I said," Don't be mad at me." Right then she glanced up into her rearview mirror and saw why I was laughing. The small version of the shopping cart sat proudly in the back of her car! Now she knew what I was laughing about, "I only borrowed it," I said, like a kid in trouble. As she was yelling at me (in a scolding way), I remembered hearing her say something about security cameras. "Why?" she asked, demanding an answer. "I only borrowed it to walk around the block with." I told her. It was sturdy and gave me my independence to take walks on my own! I would take walks in the neighborhood, but I needed to hold on to something when I did. I did not want to use my walker and told my family members I would like a stroller to push on my walks to help with my stability. Why didn't people understand that? I could not drive, and I was determined to! I had to learn to walk first, even if that meant looking like a weirdo walking around my neighborhood with a shopping cart. I Intended to teach myself how to walk with it! And I would.

I had my Life Alert and I would also carry mace with me just in case anybody thought they could mess with me. You can never be too careful nowadays. I knew it would make my family feel better. I didn't want them to worry. They had been through enough.

In the beginning, when I took a walk outside with someone, I had to hold on to the other person and could only go short distances. I really wanted to walk outside by myself and have some independence back. I could not drive a car and I was home alone a lot. So, I thought this carriage would give me my independence by allowing me to walk around the block by myself. I didn't care that I looked like a bag lady with a stolen grocery cart. It would give the neighbors something to talk about. I took it around the block a couple of times. It was great because I could put things in it. Unfortunately, it was loud and squeaky. Don't worry, like I told my sister, I was only borrowing the grocery cart, and I brought it back like I promised I would.

One day when I was out doing errands with my sister, we drove by a yard sale and I saw a baby carriage, so I had her stop. I purchased the baby carriage, and better yet, all the proceeds were going to the Jimmy Fund. I thought that making it look like there was a baby in the carriage I would look more "normal" and so I did. I rolled up and arranged a blanket to make it seem as if a baby was in there. I sometimes think to myself, if they ever knew my secret!

The Physical Therapist at the nursing home taught me to push my walker out ahead of me and walk a few steps towards it. So that's what I did with the baby carriage. I would push it out and walk towards it. As I grew better at walking, I started pushing the carriage harder. There is a very sharp corner going around my block. I would push the carriage hard there using all my might! People wouldn't see me there. It was usually very quiet. One day I pushed the baby carriage with all of my might, my strength was coming back (it must be all the weight lifting, if you call a 1lb. weight in each hand, weight lifting lol)! Right at that instant, a woman came jogging around the corner. She must have thought that I was pushing my baby into the street. Immediately, I shouted to her, holding both of my hands up to my mouth so she could hear me yelling in my newly acquired southern drawl, "There is no baby in there!" She just kept running, probably for her life! I think she thought I was a crazy woman. I am lucky the Department of Social Services didn't show up at my door. My family would have really loved that!

As I progressed my physical therapist taught me to use a cane. I hated that thing. My sister insisted that I take it when we went to the beach. I took it only to satisfy her. Walking down the crowded ramp to the beach, I waved it out in front of me saying get out of my way! Needless to say, I didn't have to take the cane with me again. But people in front of me moved!

Talking with people is what I missed the most. That's what I did best. And being a hairstylist, I had the opportunity to talk to so many people in a day. Now, I have a lot more time and more valuable things to say! I will talk to anyone that will listen. I used to wheel up to people in my wheelchair at the nursing home and ask them if they could hear me talk (because for me to speak, it took a lot of energy, and my voice was weak). If I realized they couldn't hear me, I would wheel on! Remember I was in a nursing home, so a lot of people couldn't hear me. They were hard of hearing and some of them sadly had dementia.

It was a challenge when my family took me out. I just loved to talk. I would stop and talk to anyone and everyone. First, I would tell them what happened to me and then I would say, "I gots my brains." My family would patiently wait for me.

These trips out always took a lot longer than my family had intended, no wonder nobody took me out much. Someone suggested that I say, "I still have my cognition," That sounded much better. I practiced that statement over and over again till I had it down. Occasionally I would forget mid-sentence and I would turn to my family and say, "What is that word I am supposed to use again? Thank God I have come a long way since then.

My sister would take me to a local retail hardware store to practice walking. The wide cement aisles were perfect and there were not many patrons in the lumber sections, so we had it all to ourselves. One day I needed to find a travel coffee cup while we were there. The coffee cup I carried didn't have a lid on it. My family was afraid that I would burn myself as I clumsily walked with the hot coffee in my walker around my house. We had to find a coffee cup with a lid that fit in a Keurig machine. I asked one of the employees if they sold any coffee cups with lids? He said yes and showed me where they were. The cups were fine. The only problem was that they didn't fit in the Keurig machine. They were too tall. The salesman told us that he had a cup that fit his Keurig and how great it was. He offered to give it to me. I kept saying no but he insisted, so I decided to take the cup. While he was cleaning the cup out, I took off my sweatshirt because it was warm, and he noticed the Life Alert hanging from my neck. It was a regular fixture for me and I forgot that I even wore it. "What is that...are you taping me?" he asked. I think he thought he was being taped for a reality show. I briefly explained what had happened to me and why it was there. I bet he never felt so good about giving a coffee cup away to help another person. This gesture, I will never forget! When we returned again, we stopped and got him a cup of coffee. I try to pay it forward! Pay it forward is an expression for describing the beneficiary of a good deed repaying it to others instead of to the original benefactor.

One time I had forgotten a client's last name. So, I asked her sister, who was also an excellent client of mine, what her sister's last name was. I have a hard time remembering my former client's names. My brain injury has affected that, even without having a brain injury, I still couldn't remember all of their names. So, I sent her a message via Facebook messenger asking for her sister's last name. She returned my message with, "Backoff." I was so upset that I actually cried and shut my computer off. Later that day, I sent her a reply, saying that I was so sorry and that I would not ever bother her again. She immediately sent me back a reply saying that she loved me and explained that her sister's last name is actually Backoff. What?? Oh yes that's right it is her last name. Ok I remember now, and I will never forget it again!

I went to the grocery store with my sister another time and this time I went inside with her. I pushed myself to go. Starting out I would go with my sister following her around. Everything was a teaching moment. I saw a bag of small donuts, so I took them and ate a couple around the store as she shopped. When we got to the checkout, my sister asked me where the donuts were that I was eating. I couldn't remember so I told her that I put them back. Let's just say with me around there is never a dull moment! The brain hemorrhage had left me with no inhibition, just like a child would take something and not know any better, that was me. I had to relearn these things.

I exercised and tried to do everything I was told to. My sister suggested we go walking on a local college campus that was not far from our home, so we would go there every evening. It was a great obstacle course. It had a hill, stairs, walkways and grassy areas. These were all good challenges for me. It was mid-spring, and we noticed that on most of the tree-lined areas, which were where the walkway paths were, the trees were loaded with caterpillars, They were also all over the walkways. We had walked quiet a distance without noticing how bad the caterpillars were. It got worse the further we went. We were in too deep now to turn around. "Just don't look." I remember her telling me! Crunch, crunch. The crunch is all I heard! I'll admit it did make my walking faster. I just remember praying that I didn't fall! Needless to say, that was the most disgusting walk I have ever taken.

When we were back at the car, we looked across the parking lot and saw the track. "That is where we are going to walk from now on" I said. The track was perfect. It had professional lines painted on it, which helped me walk straight as I tended to drift to the left when I walked. It would keep me focused on walking straight. There was a sand pit which was great for my balance and to prepare me for the beach. It also had a big cushion that was used for the vault jump, and we used it to stretch out and do exercises on. I also balanced on the painted lines in the field like a sobriety test, not that I have ever had one of these tests. We would count how many steps I could go until I fell off the line. Every day I tried to push myself a little further. The track was a great idea.

My sister is a Social Worker in a nursing facility, so she had some good ideas. She suggested that I go to the local senior center exercise class. So off I went. If you were a citizen of the town, you could use the services provided. They also had a van service that would take you locally where you needed to go. Seeing that I didn't have my license at the time and everyone worked, I utilized the van service. I didn't want to inconvenience anyone. I had already done that and although a little wobbly I was becoming more and more physically independent. So, the van it was. It would pick me up and take me to the Senior Center for exercise class. It was all older people that were trying their best to remain active Remember use it or lose it. They were very kind and accepting of me. They were very compassionate. I think that they understood my problems much better than people my own age. A lot of them had been through hardships and have had health issues themselves. This was a very supportive group and we liked each other. During exercise class, we laughed a lot and the instructors had to keep us in our place. There was one elderly gentleman who everybody loved. He would address all of us as "girlfriend" because he could not remember our names. One day I forgot his name, so I called him "boyfriend". We all laughed and again, we all had a good time. We enjoyed this gentleman so much. It is amazing how one person can make a big difference. It is all in your attitude.

Our elders have so much to offer and from what I have seen we don't value them as we should. They seem to be a burden or a chore for a lot of people. My eyes have been made wide open now, and it's shameful! Other cultures are much better at taking care of their elders. They evidently know what's important!

•••• 9 ••••

A REMINDER

"In the End, we will remember not the words of our enemies, but the silence of our friends"
—**Martin Luther King, Jr**

ALL I WANTED was to be normal again. The AVM rupture was a hard slap in the face, and it stung like hell. I Thought I was invincible, but as it turns out, not so much. There is a good quote that I think of often:

When life knocks you down, calmly get back up, smile, and very politely say, "You hit like a bitch."

Awhile before the brain bleed (AVM) occurred, I had asked myself, "Is this all there is?" I was spoiled; and I knew it. I had everything pretty much that I ever wanted. I had a great life. I was very fortunate. However, I had received a harsh answer. In experiencing the aftermath of an AVM rupture, I learned that NO... this is not all that there is! My life isn't over. I'm taking a new path, and it has just begun.

I didn't actually hear it. I learned the lesson loud and clear. Yes, It was made perfectly clear to me. Listening to the silence, I did a complete turnaround, a 360. Now I'm here to share it with you. I wish that people's insides were as good as they looked on the outside. We definitely have this backward. Life is not all about how you look. It's about how you act and contribute to society. What kind of person you are, is what really matters! Is it always someone else's problem? That seems to be some people's solution. Look out for number one and it's too bad for anyone else. We have become a very desensitized and selfish society. I was, unfortunately, one of "those people." Fortunately for me, I got to see the other side. Yes, let me repeat myself. Fortunate is how I now feel!

I know that I am very lucky and at times I don't always act that way. I am very fortunate to even be here with the ones that I love, even though I have a hard time showing it. I have so much to be thankful for. I am not physically sick, and I have no pain. That in and of itself is a miracle! Lucky doesn't even begin to describe what we all went through. I am very GRATEFUL!

People move on, run away from you. Yes, sometimes they run like hell! You just don't see or hear from them anymore. At least, this happened to me. I learned this well after I returned home. I had been away for a tough long three months. The crisis had been over for others, probably when they heard that I was not at death's door anymore. Some people were perhaps relieved! I should say released! It made them feel as if they didn't have to carry the burden anymore. I was going to be fine they thought, so no problem for them.

I call Facebook, FAKEBOOK, because people only post the really good stuff like there's no bad. Essentially it looks to others that you live a flawless life, which is untrue for everyone! Picture perfect or so it seems, but I know the truth, it is not. Everyone has difficulties in their lives, they just don't want to show that. This is so fake.. Facebook has you call acquaintances friends. Probably because acquaintances sound cold. I'm sure it's a marketing thing. Acquaintances know how to delete you. It's easy for them. Sadly, to be honest, I would have probably done this myself.

Facebook was like a lifeline for me. It was difficult for me to leave the house and communicate with people, and this kept me informed of what was going on. It helped pass the day. Unfortunately, sometimes it was difficult, as I would see my friends going out, having fun, posting pictures on Facebook, and leaving me with the feeling of being left behind, forgotten. Life was going on without me.

Now, I watch and learn. This teaches me a lot. Once you stop and put yourself in other people's shoes, you can somewhat imagine how they feel! I don't say anything now unless I see it with my own eyes. I might choose not to say something. I've learned to keep a lot of things to myself now. My filter is coming back! Trust seems to be an issue for me where it wasn't before. You have to be very careful whom you trust. I learned this the hard way. There's a song written by Garth Brooks titled, The Dance - *"Yes, my life is better left to chance. I could have missed the pain, but I would have missed the dance."*

I was isolated by this monster called an AVM rupture! Yes, I had my computer and it was useful to go on some social media platforms, but what I needed was real people to talk to, not electronics. This only increases loneliness. People need real human contact and not electronic devices regularly. THINK. A friendly voice means so much more than digital text. Get sick, and you'll find out!

I assume that most people don't know what to say to someone in a crisis. Guess what? Nobody does! All that anybody wants is your presence. Just knowing that they are not alone. There is this skill called "listening." I have yet to master it myself! If they don't want to talk, just be there for a little bit. Just let them know you are there for them, and you are still their friend or acquaintance! If you are there for them, you're a friend. This is why I love this quote: "Actions speak a lot louder than words." This now has depth...It is so very very true!

We are just in need of a little bit of your time, even if that means driving around in the car with you while you do your errands. It's hard for you. We know that. Put yourselves in the other person's shoes for a moment. (oh no, they're too small and they hurt) sorry. I don't want to make things uncomfortable for you! Here put on these comfy slippers. They feel better anyway and look good too! Yes, I'm being facetious! As I am writing this, I can hear my mother saying put your filter on! I was left alone, quite often.

Most people my age have to go to work, families to care for and they have their own lives to live. I understand that and no I don't want a pity-party or my ass kissed. Yes, I was told that via a very hurtful text. All I would like and very much appreciate is an hour of somebody's time once in a while, with the people that I choose to be around. Is that too much to ask? Evidently, it is. Oh, I know? Poor me Right? No poor you! Your loss, I would probably be the best friend you would have ever had (I don't want to offend anyone, now that's funny!). I take your feelings into consideration what about mine. THINK! I miss work and everything about it, especially the social aspect. Who would ever imagine that I would be saying that? I really liked all my clients. It took me years to find and keep them. I feel like I suddenly up and left them. It's like coming home, your house is empty and, your husband left, taking everything with him. This is the only way I can explain it.

Here comes another saying, "What you give out you get back." I don't know who wrote that, but there is a song called, "You Get What You Give" by the New Radicals. Well, I guess I was given everything that I gave out in the friend department. That's why I say that there is a big difference between friends and acquaintances! Now I am different, but I'm only better. I don't understand why people don't know that? I am only a better person from having this AVM rupture! I have learned so much, and I have been given a second chance that I do not intend to waste.

After my AVM I had nothing to do. I listened to a lot of music and started writing. However, when I did get the chance to talk to somebody, I would talk their ear off in my slow southern drawl, and half of it I'm sure they didn't understand. This is where the hairstylist in me came out, evidently, now I had a lot to say!

This is how I got people's attention. By swearing! It is like verbal punctuation to me! If you want to get someone's attention swear! My mother has told me that it lowers me. I know this is true, but it is difficult not to swear. It's like saying no to that fabulous dessert. I try to refrain. *Restraint*, now that's another subject for another time.

Hurt, resentment, pain, yes; I have experienced it all. Although, I choose to see the good things that I have in my life, my husband, daughter, parents and sister, and some family and friends.

Somebody I thought was a good friend, turned out not to be. I know that I am now somewhat different, but still the same only better. I just needed and wanted a friend. This unfortunately happens to many other survivors, also. During my recovery I found myself somewhat alone. I wish some of my friends and family educated themselves about brain injury. When I did not have my filter and said some inappropriate or hurtful things, it was not intentional. They did not understand that everything was and continues to be an effort for me and others with this affliction. Some people treated me as though I was a child, and I just wanted to be treated normal. I would try to do some things. Some friends thought they were being helpful by taking over, but this made me feel inadequate. I did not like feeling like an invalid. If I was going to relearn and get better; I had to do things for myself. If you want to help someone with a brain injury, it is important to educate yourself. It is important for the survivor to be surround with people that will lift them up!

However, all I wanted now was friends that I could learn from. Yes, everyone has something they can teach you, I know that. I wanted to educate myself on new things. I wanted to expand my knowledge and awareness. In my old life I was just interested in my image, shopping, impressing people etc. You get the picture. I now took the mask off and found out what was really important.

The people I know seem quite content in their lives. I feel, as I'm sure most survivors do, like starting all over again. I have a new lease on life and I am determined to make the best of it!

I do things now that I would have never done in my old life. No one would have ever believed that I would get up early on a cold, rainy Saturday morning to volunteer to pick up other people's trash. Get my nails dirty? I don't think so. Write a book? I would hardly ever read a book. Exercise at the Senior Center. Exercise Never! I have definitely changed for the better.

I can count my true friends on one hand. My family is so important. I am so very grateful! I have read stories of people that don't have families or have disowned their family. This is very sad to me, but its reality. "THINK." People with a brain injury cannot do it alone. You need to have a team around you of people you can trust with your life. This doesn't come easy. Don't be afraid to ask for help even though this was very difficult for me and still is. Asking for help is not my strong point.

When my injury first happened, my family set up a "Sheri update page" on Facebook, which was for close friends and family, to let them know what was going on with me. When I first came home, they posted that I would need help with my exercises and asked for volunteers. This worked out well as different family members and friends helped me and made it fun and interesting. I also enjoyed their visits and had something to look forward to.

They all had different ideas and exercises to do with me. Some of the ideas were very creative. My Uncle would tell me to reach up and hit the top of the doorways this helped stretch out my arm and helped with balance. I forgot to mention that I had a had a frozen shoulder, which sometimes happens after a stroke.

I went to a chiropractor who tried to help me with my frozen shoulder. It was helpful, but I was still having trouble raising my arm. I then went to an orthopedist, (who was very handsome by the way) he discussed my options to fix my shoulder. I then asked him, "Who do you love?" He looked at me quizzically and replied, "Tom Brady". So, I then asked him to treat me like him. He said "Oh, I should have said my wife and mother." We laughed. I got my point across. He gave me two Cortisone shots one in the front and one back of my shoulder. I was given an exercise plan to follow. Now my shoulder is fine. I can lift my arm up over my head.

As I was starting to slowly get better, I felt as though I had been shunned by some so-called friends, Mother's that I wanted to fit in with, people that lived in my town. They all had their own reasons for not accepting me. I would just have to deal with it. I was never put into a situation like this, having to be accepted by others and not having anything to offer except friendship. I am sure much of the way I was treated was my own fault. I had not been a leader, I had been a follower. I know this now. I just assumed this would never happen to me. You might know what assume means, *it makes an ASS out of you and me!* I am a strong person, and now it was time to prove it.

Overall, I do have a great support system. It was very heartwarming when one of my old friends heard the tragedy my family and I had encountered. She and her salon had a

Cut*A*Thon Fundraiser for me. They contacted several of the hairdressers that I had worked with over the years and had a day devoted to me (knowing at the time that I must have been drowning in bills). So yes, I do have some true, caring friends! Most people tend to have their hearts in the right place.

I had another friend voluntarily start a Go-Fund-Me page, and I very much appreciated her thoughtfulness and everyone who contributed.

This also brings me to a gift that I was given by a friend for my birthday. A ring that is meant to be worn on your middle finger. I love it. I wear it all the time. It has more than one meaning, (if you get what I mean.) I am so happy that some days just knowing that I have on this ring is enough! I wear this ring a lot especially when I know I'll be driving. Nowadays, others on the road can be rather rude and in such a hurry that they tend not to have consideration for other people driving on the road. Instead of giving them the middle finger and putting my life at risk. I wear my ring and it's my own private joke. I say to myself "Hmm, if they only knew my secret."

This town that I live in is beautiful. The people here, well let's put it this way, I was just like them before my AVM. I was very wrapped up in my own life. Always concerned about looking good and having the best of everything. But that life was not what I wanted anymore. I now see things clearer and I really couldn't care less about monetary things and things that seem trivial.

I feel I'm fortunate because I am very optimistic, and I try to see the best in everyone. I even try to look for the good in everything, even if it sucks! I appreciate the good things even more now, because I choose to make a conscious effort to do so. Even though I have had a good life, there is always room for improvement. I'm not a holy roller, but I do believe in God. My relationship with Him is private, as I'm sure, it is for most people.

••••10••••

#AWARENESS

"We are only as blind as we want to be."
—Maya Angelou

WHEN I ARRIVED home, I didn't use a computer for a long time (about a year). I had too many other things to do, appointments to keep, medications to take, Dr appointments, visiting nurses, physical therapist, speech therapist, neurologists, blood pressure, cognitive exercises, regular exercise, showers and the list goes on and on.

Now I am an expert in one thing, and that's being a warrior of a brain Arteriovenous Malformation (AVM) rupture. I have lived it. I watched a lot of politics. Actually, it was all I watched. I wanted to get smarter and I liked the way they talked. I, however, didn't always like what was being said. I could think for myself, that's right this is a miracle! I have been very affected by this, and I am determined to educate people.

I relearned how to use the computer, and I am still learning by the way. I wanted to learn more about what had happened to me and how to get better. I looked up brain aneurysms after I had been home for a while to educate myself. These sites are not only educational but also supportive. I found the Brain Aneurysm Foundation (BAF) on the computer. Their site is beneficial and informative. A very helpful resource to anyone who has been afflicted by a brain aneurysm or an AVM. This organization is the closest one to my heart for many reasons! They do a lot of great work. The Brain Aneurysm Foundation is a patient resource directory for individuals and families affected by brain aneurysms and is constantly updated with the newest information. These are such wonderful people. The Brain Aneurysm Foundation is a globally recognized leader in brain aneurysm awareness, education, support, advocacy, and research funding.

There are also other beneficial sites online as well. There seems to be a lot more available now because they are learning more about this new frontier called YOUR BRAIN!

One subject that I want to talk about is the lack of family and friends staying informed on this issue, just because you can't see it doesn't mean it's not there. People that have been afflicted with this illness are not lazy and using this as an excuse! Believe me they are doing the best they can and they probably really need your help and understanding.

There is such a thing as Neuro-Fatigue. People describe Neuro-Fatigue as an overwhelming tiredness or complete exhaustion. Fatigue can affect you physically and emotionally. When I first came home, I would go to bed early and take naps throughout the day. I would get fatigued easily after doing one simple chore. It has taken me a long time to regain my stamina and I am still working on it.

What others don't understand is that it is difficult for me to talk. It uses up a lot of my energy. Think of energy like this. (I heard this from Amy Zellmer.) Amy is a writer and a nationally known TBI advocate. Think of energy as money. You get five dollars a day. It takes three dollars to wash and dry your hair. How will you use the rest of your energy (money) on the rest of your day?

Some of the simplest things affect me now. going inside to outside, temperature, sunlight, and even the wind. Even standing up takes effort for me now. Going to a store is overwhelming to a brain injured person. Everything on the shelves is sensory overstimulation, or what is called "Flooding." This occurs after a brain injury because the brain's 'filters' no longer work properly.

I have experienced "flooding." I especially feel this in stores. All the different products, colors, shapes, sound, light, and motion around us daily bother a lot of TBI and brain aneurysm patients. Personally, it took me a long time before I was ready to go into a store. I would go to the local pharmacy with my walker and would attempt to walk the perimeter. This store was chosen by my family because it had seats at the rear of the store to sit in. The first time I walked in this store I felt so overwhelmed that I could only stay in there for a few minutes. I remember I could not look around because there was too much stimulation. The music, light, noises, people and all of the different colors on the shelves that all blended together were too much for me. I would primarily keep my head down and look at my feet when walking around the store with my trusty walker. It took me a long time to overcome this obstacle. I do love to shop, but I still have some flooding which is improving slowly with time.

I also know that it's common for people to die from a brain bleed. People die from a AVM or aneurysm ruptures frequently. This is honestly so very sad and often preventable if caught early. Every individual case is different. I can't stress this enough. Every part of the brain controls different functions, so the residuals from a brain bleed are very different depending on which part of the brain was affected.

I know that if I lived in constant pain and had different deficits, I might feel a lot different physically and mentally than I do today. Everyone's recovery is so very different. Take one step forward every day to better yourself, and to have a better outcome. THINK baby steps! You have to get up, get dressed, show up, and be accountable! Do things that you're uncomfortable doing! Who cares? You do! Get comfortable being uncomfortable. Sometimes you need to put yourself out there and do different things! This is also very good for your brain. The Medical staff didn't give me or my family much information about brain aneurysms or recovery, with the exception of what medications to take and when, probably because I went from one facility to another and wasn't at the time capable enough to handle it correctly. Hopefully, this will change. Right now there isn't much available to brain injury survivors. This is a new frontier. Technology and awareness are slowly and surely making a change. New advances are giving patients and caregivers information about what they need so desperately! I am most grateful for this as I'm sure all of the Brain Injury community is!

We look fine, and you can't physically see the disorder. Now you just might get a glimpse as to what goes on in my life and many others! Just knowing that I am truly very lucky, and I don't have many of the health problems that afflict others! For this, I will always be GRATEFUL. Some survivors, however, don't feel this way. Some suffer from mental illness, pain, apathy, cognitive problems, memory issues, sleep issues, headaches, survivor's guilt, PTSD, depression and the list, goes unfortunately, on.

I read a lot of survivor's stories, and it's very unfortunate. There is so much to this, that is why I am trying to bring this to your attention! Being a brain AVM survivor as well, I feel as though I am equipped with a lot of knowledge. This is why the Brain Aneurysm Foundation (BAF) is so critical, as are the others that bring awareness to this subject. They fight this fight every day! We are entering a new frontier. The medical community is learning new things about the brain every day through technology. This is why they are saving so many lives, Mine being one of them, and so many, others. The brain is a very complex organ that we, unfortunately, take for granted. Well, at least I did, before being thrown into this awful situation, I have learned a lot about the brain. There is a brain aneurysm rupturing every 18 minutes. Ruptured brain aneurysms are fatal in about 40% of cases. Of those who survive, about 66% suffer some permanent neurological deficit. Approximately 15% of patients with aneurysmal subarachnoid hemorrhage (SAH) die before reaching the hospital.

People with unruptured aneurysms often feel like they are walking around with a ticking time bomb in their head.

What is an aneurysm? An aneurysm is an abnormal widening or ballooning of a part of an artery due to weakness in the wall of the blood vessel. An aneurysm is a blood-filled bulge of a blood vessel. It is usually caused by disease or the walls of the blood vessel become weak. Aneurysms typically happen in arteries at the base of the brain and in the aorta (the main artery coming out of the heart) — this is an aortic aneurysm. This bulge in a blood vessel can burst or break open and cause the person to die at any time. The larger an aneurysm becomes, the more likely it is to burst. Aneurysms can often be treated.

A ruptured aneurysm releases blood into the spaces around the brain, called a *subarachnoid hemorrhage* (SAH) is life threatening with a 50% risk of death. Blood in the subarachnoid space increases pressure on the brain, a complication that can sometimes occur 5 to 10 days after aneurysm rupture is vasospasm.

A subarachnoid hemorrhage is bleeding into the subarachnoid space (the space between the arachnoid and the pia mater). ("Subarachnoid" means "under the arachnoid.") Because the subarachnoid space holds cerebrospinal fluid, bleeding here makes the blood mix into the cerebrospinal fluid. The blood irritates the brain and spinal cord and causes symptoms like a horrible headache and a stiff neck.

TBI the definition: Traumatic Brain Injury (TBI) is an insult to the brain, not of a degenerative or congenital nature, but caused by an external physical force that may produce a diminished or altered state of consciousness, which results in an impairment of cognitive abilities or physical functioning. There is no known cure for this. Brain injuries take some years to heal and some last a lifetime. All brain affliction is different depending on what part of the brain is affected. The doctors are only human and some things they just don't know. The brain seems to be the next big frontier. Due to the complexity of it! I now understand why. Recovery is complicated to predict. Sleep is vital for brain injury patients as this is when your brain heals. Exercise is also very important! The more you do, the better the outcome. You have the idea that the hospital is where you rest, well some of that is true. When I was transferred to Spaulding Rehabilitation Hospital that all changed! Yeah, it's named that for a reason I found out (Rehabilitation Hospital)!

•••• 11 ••••

COMPASSION

"Never look down on anybody unless you're helping them up."
—Jesse Jackson

PEOPLE WITH BRAIN injury often suffer in silence. We are unique in the fact that you cannot see it! If you wore a cast or are confined to a wheelchair, you would be aware that something was wrong, but not with most brain injury patients unless they tell you and make you aware of their condition. People think that I'm either deaf because of the way I talk or drunk because of my balance issues. Who am I kidding? I would have thought that too! Looking at people I learned that they only tell you what they want you to know. We create an image around ourselves for protection. It's a false sense of protection. We all care too much about what other people think of us. It is time to *wash off the fake*.

My husband once said to me before this happened, "I wouldn't want to be stuck on a deserted island with you." I thought about that one day recently. Replying to myself, I bet he would want to be stuck on an island with me now! You don't know how lucky you are to have a warrior survivor in your life! I like this definition of a warrior: A person who endures a lot more than others physically and mentally. I have personally learned so much from this AVM rupture.

We need more compassion in the world. I don't say much unless I see it with my own eyes and I have seen it lacking, first hand. I am talking to you. Look at yourself and tell me what you see? Families even lack in this area toward one another. Everyone has feelings and problems. They may be fighting battles you know nothing about. I found out a lot of people are not as compassionate as they want you to think they are. They are not doing this intentionally (or maybe they are). They just run away as far as they can get. When there's a fire, run! However, don't come back for warmth, and whatever you do don't help to put it out. For the most part, it's not what they do, but what they don't do. When you don't do anything, you are part of the problem. I have learned this the hard way, but the key here is I learned.

Some people think it's all about them and who has the best stuff. Sadly, we have taught this to our children. We want them to have a better life than we did (which wasn't so bad). We created material-minded, uncompassionate people. They don't have much to look forward to. We have tried to give them everything they need to make themselves comfortable. In doing so, we are going to be in trouble when they have to see for themselves what the real world holds. This is sad, very sad but true from my point of view. I'm not saying that I didn't do some of this myself. Regretfully I did, but back then I thought I was doing the right thing. Sometimes it takes "tough love." That is hard to do. I was told this by my father when I was a little girl, "The only person that you can depend on is yourself." This stuck with me. Others can try to help, but ultimately it is up to you. I know that every situation is different, and I see both sides.

Maybe educating yourself on the subject of aneurysms or AVM might help! Or whatever the person's crisis is. This is what I mean about educating yourself. Some people just don't take the time. Educate yourself even just a little bit. This shows that you care! It's not like you have cancer or anything (yes this actually was said to someone that suffered a traumatic brain injury). Believe me it's just as bad! This has happened to others. This is why I say THINK! Sometimes we don't need words, maybe being there is good enough. You are a gift, especially to someone who is sick. They probably aren't exposed to people that much. I know it's uncomfortable for you, just imagine how uncomfortable it is for them. This once again brings me to how actions speak louder. This is where and when people show you what you really mean to them. I listened to the silence and experienced the good In some people. My personal experience was both. Like life, there's no good without bad.

The longer my recovery took, the quieter it became. Well, at least this was a portion of my experience. My parents and their spouses were always there for me, and I knew that. Most of them were growing older and weary. I'm sure a lot of others are experiencing this also. It is hard to ask someone for help during the bad times. We just take this for granted and assume that they will be there. I was sadly somewhat mistaken. I was grateful and lucky that some people were there for me, doing what they could to get me back on my feet, Which I will always be grateful for (I was told that I pushed a lot of people away, which is normal by the way). I didn't want them to see me weak and vulnerable. This was hard enough, so why hurt others in the process, I thought. Now I know what they mean when they say, you're lucky if you have a couple of people that you can really count on in your life. Yes, this is very true!

People with an illness, don't want to be thought of as helpless and weak, never-mind being seen as needy! They all say, call me if you need anything. It is kind of like a guy asking you for your phone number hoping that he will call, but never does. This is somewhat of a kind gesture, but most people won't call. This is too difficult for them, emotionally appearing weak! We're not programmed to be needy. We would rather do it ourselves! Here's an idea, just do a task for them without asking. (yes, here I'm being a wise ass!) Sometimes you have to be forceful. Some people are stubborn! But I am sure they will be very appreciative! Do some cleaning, buy some groceries, mow the lawn! I know it's work and money. The two things people have a very hard time with is giving! The social aspect is very important. Yes, social interaction is great for your health! Yes, both parties can benefit from this! Yes, I know you're very busy, aren't we all?

The caregivers especially need support. Most of the time they are forgotten. They do their best to care for the brain injured person. They often need to do everything: hygiene, laundry, food, medications, appointments, rides, cleaning, bills.... The caregiver needs to manage all of that, including their own lives. No one wants to think of ever becoming a caregiver. We need to support the people that do this very important work! It is imperative. Maybe not to you, but to somebody else it can be life or death. The quality of your life depends on others. Now, this is a very big responsibility! Waiting on somebody else to do what no one wants to. This is to some, a privilege. Being a caregiver is one of the hardest jobs you can ever take on. It's hard enough to care physically for someone else, but financially it can be challenging! This is why a lot of people tend to walk, or maybe I should say run. Yes, some of them even run away!

I have personally learned so much from this happening to me. I want to give back what I learned! I'm extremely grateful that I can learn and grow. This is what I want for you, too! Unfortunately, this experience happens to most people at some point in their lives. They get sick. We just don't want to think about this never mind talk about it.

I find a lot of this information very overwhelming, so I want to provide you with some basic, helpful knowledge that I have learned along the way. I want to end this book by stating that there is help out there, although you have to be willing to look and find information that will fit your needs. As I have stated before, every brain injury is different. I know that to you and your family your life is the most important! I want to see you heal. You have to try to get better for yourself. NOBODY else is responsible for your life! You have to get up and try! Given the right conditions, the brain can overcome adversity, so that some function is recovered. Try to take your life back into your own hands. I know that's what you want, and I'm not saying it will be easy. I'm saying it will be worth it!

I want you to know one more very crucial piece of information that I have definitely learned throughout this experience, as I told select senators on Capitol Hill. This disease has been physically, emotionally, and financially devastating to many.

My sister and I participated with the Brain Aneurysm Advocacy Day. This event is held every year by the Brain Aneurysm Foundation. A delegation composed of brain aneurysm survivors, family members, advocates and medical professionals from around the country participate every year for Congressional Advocacy Day. The effort set forth is to raise awareness of brain aneurysm disease and to seek support for Ellie's Law.

Ellie Helton, Lisa Colagrossi, Teresa Anne Lawrence, and Jennifer Sedney Focused Research Act of Ellie's Law

This bill authorizes appropriations for the National Institute of Neurological Disorders and Stroke to conduct or support research on unruptured brain aneurysms in a patient population diversified by age, sex, and race.

••••12••••

TIPS

"Be a Rainbow in someone else's Cloud"
—Maya Angelou

Basic tips I learned going through a Brain Hemorrhage. Some of these tips are for the patient, some for caregivers/ friends, and some general tips for all:

1. Take care of your body. It is your home and the only one you have.
2. Always be kind to people. You never really know what someone is going through.
3. Offer to help people you don't know. Actions speak louder than words and what you give out you get back. (I'm a big believer in this now!) Don't just say you are going to do something. Actually, just do it. Everyone has a gift within themselves. Everyone has something

to give even if it's being a friend to someone. This is the most important of all.

4. Join a local volunteer group, religious organizations, town organizations such as food pantry or the library. Look on the computer for volunteer groups in your area.

5. It is true, life does begin at the end of your comfort zone. Get comfortable being uncomfortable mentally, emotionally, and physically. Do something you would usually not do.

6. It is better to work together as a team with family, friends, doctors and caregivers; you will accomplish more.

7. Be around people that will lift you up! Let go of people that will pull you down.

8. The brain takes a very long time to heal. The saying, use it or lose it, fits brain injuries quite well. Take classes. The more you use the brain, the better! Once again this is true! THINK!

9. People don't walk. They RUN! Think of a car accident on the highway and people rubbernecking. They all slow down to look and speed off after they have seen what happened. Don't be a rubbernecker. Be a friend.

10. Life is hard for everyone. There is no good without bad, but this is what living is about! Views will change, meanings will change, purposes will change. You will realize at the end of your life, people don't care about the material, fake stuff that you may have once thought was important to show the world.

11. There is no easy path to take. All end up being hard in different ways, but the one that looks hard in the beginning is the one with the biggest payoff, emotionally and physically.

12. The only person you really truly can depend on is yourself. If you're lucky, some of your family members

or really great friends will be there for you. I found seniors are good to one another. They help each other, probably because they have lived through hardships. We should all learn from that!

13. One thing I can guarantee: we are all going to get old and are quite possibly have an illness. It is going to be hard. Please plan for this. Have important items in order. It will make your life and your loved ones lives a little bit easier.

14. Be social! This is so good for you and your brain. Try really hard not to gossip. It can come back to bite you!

15. Join a support group. They are online as well as in a lot of hospitals.

16. Silence can be bad. It is best to let your feelings be known. Talking it out is best for everyone. I resented everyone's silence. People stayed away in some instances because they didn't know what to say. For some, seeing me was once a reminder of their own mortality.

17. Try educating yourself on the subject at hand, even if it's just a little. You will be much more respected for this. Just because a person does not show any physical signs doesn't mean that they have not been affected. Talk to them, include them, don't isolate them, encourage them.

18. Say "Hi" to people. Engage people in conversation, show them you are friendly. It will lift their spirits. People don't acknowledge others anymore unless they are trying to sell something and are told to acknowledge you. Go into a store and you will see what I mean!

19. Smile! I do this a lot especially when I don't feel good about something or I am uncomfortable. This tells my mind that I like it. There is always room for improvement, so try to smile. It's not hard. "We need this social connection". I'm not saying to be a weirdo about it. Don't go around smiling and saying hi to

everyone! Do it casually and you will see the benefits and notice other people at the same time.

20. Keep a calendar! It will help you and your support team know who, what, and where? A to-do list it also helpful!

21. The family of the patient needs to eat. Often they have spent numerous hours at the hospital or commuting to and from. If you decide to help someone by dropping off a meal, a simple home cooked meal will warm their soul instead of fast food.

22. Once the patient is home, take up all scatter rugs in the house to help prevent trips and falls.

23. Meditation can be helpful: reduces depression, tiredness, and fatigue, It can also improve balance, attention, concentration and emotions.

24. Drink a lot of water. It is good for your brain.

25. A Medical Alert necklace or pendant can be very helpful when the person is left alone and may have a medical emergency.

26. Get a pill box to keep the medication organized.

27. Take notes during doctor's appointments. It is always good to have someone go with you to the doctor's office.

28. Take pictures of your journey. Then you can see your progress.

29. There will be difficult days, but don't give up. Tomorrow is a new day. Play brain games, do crossword puzzles, word search, read, etc...

30. Exercise, Exercise, Exercise. If you don't use it, you will lose it!

31. Diet is very important for your brain, so eat well and take your vitamins. Your gut is associated with your brain.

32. Social media is great communication and social tool. However, don't isolate yourself. Mix it up!

33. You're going to be creating a new path for yourself, don't let things happen. Make things happen!
34. Use of Emojis help to express how you are feeling.
35. Work on your personal growth! You are stronger than you THINK!

Warning signs of an aneurysm

(This is copied from the Brain Aneurysm Foundation
https://www.bafound.org**)**

Unruptured brain aneurysms are typically completely asymptomatic. These aneurysms are typically small in size, usually less than one half inch in diameter. However, large unruptured aneurysms can occasionally press on the brain or the nerves stemming out of the brain and may result in various neurological symptoms. Ruptured brain aneurysms usually result in a subarachnoid hemorrhage (SAH), which is defined as bleeding into the subarachnoid space. When blood escapes into the space around the brain, it can cause sudden symptoms. Any individual experiencing some or all of the following symptoms, regardless of age, should undergo immediate and careful evaluation by a physician:

-Localized Headache
-Dilated pupils
-Blurred or double vision

-Pain above and behind eye
-Weakness and numbness
-Sudden severe headache, the worst headache of your life
-Loss of consciousness
-Nausea/Vomiting
-Stiff Neck
-Sudden blurred or double vision
-Sudden pain above/behind the eye or difficulty seeing
-Sudden change in mental status/awareness
-Sudden trouble walking or dizziness
-Sudden weakness and numbness
-Sensitivity to light (photophobia)
-Seizure
-Drooping eyelid
-Difficulty speaking

"We can watch life from the sidelines, or actively partici-
pate…. either we let self doubt and feelings of inadequacy
prevent us from realizing our potential, or embrace the fact
that when we turn our attention away from ourselves,
our potential is limitless"
—Christopher Reeve

My Favorite Song List

The reason for this song list is because while at Home recovering, I listened often to these empowering songs. (I interpreted some of them differently.) Here is a list of songs that all have great meaning to me in some way. I hope you can relate and find meaning in them for yourself. Music is profoundly powerful !

In Alphabetical order

Adele: a million years ago
Christina Aguilera : fighter
Sara Bareilles : Many the miles/ Brave/ she used to be mine
Natasha Bedingfield : unwritten
Black eyed peas : I gotta feeling
Mary J. Blige: Family Affair
Colbie Caillat : Try / I'm never gonna let you down
Andrea Day : Rise up
Black eyed peas : I gotta feeling
Blurry : Puddle of mudd
Alessia Cara : scars to your beautiful
Mariah Carey : Make it happen
Colbie Caillat : try/ I'm never gonna let you down

Kenny Chesney : Don't blink
Kelly Clarkson : Miss independent / Breakaway
Miley Cyrus: The climb
Destiny's child : Survivor
Duffy : I'm scared
Fergie : Big girls don't cry
Florence and the machine : The dog days are over
Garth Brooks : The dance
Great big world : Say something I'm giving up on you
Green Day : Time of your life
Imagine Dragons : Radioactive / Believer / Thunder
Michael Jackson : You are not alone/Man in the mirror /Smile
Kasha : praying
Alicia Keys : girl on fire
Linkin park : In the end
LP/ lost on you
Mandisa : Overcomer
Bruno Mars : Uptown funk
Matchbox twenty : Unwell / Push
Idina Menzel : let it go
Imagine Dragons:
Nickelback : If today was your last day / If everyone cared
New radicals : you get what you give
No doubt : Don't speak
Nico and Vinz : Am I wrong
Katy perry : Roar / Rise / Firework
Christina Perri : A Thousand years
Pharrell williams : Happy
Pink : Just like fire / So what / Try/ Raise your glass/
Perfect lyrics
Queen : We are the champions
Rachel platten : Fight song / Stand by you
Rascal Flatts : My wish for you / What hurts the most
Rocky : Eye of the tiger
Sia : Elastic heart / Titanium

Smash mouth : All star
The Fray : Over my head
The greatest showman : This is me
Justin Timberlake : Can't stop the feeling
Carrie Underwood with Ludicrous : The champion
Wiz Khalifa : See you again
Yael Naïm : New soul
3 Doors down : When I'm gone /
It's not my time / kryptonite

Glossary

(This is copied from the Brain Aneurysm Foundation and the Webster's dictionary
https://www.bafound.org**)**

Aneurysm: An aneurysm occurs when part of an artery wall weakens, allowing it to balloon out or widen abnormally. If it gets too large, it can rupture. The bleeding can be life-threatening. Large aneurysms should be treated. The causes of aneurysms are sometimes unknown. Some may be congenital, meaning a person is born with them.

Angiogram: detects blockages using X-rays taken. This produces an image that can help your doctor find blockages or other abnormalities in the blood vessels of your head and neck. Blockages or abnormalities can lead to a stroke or bleeding in the brain.

Aphasia: A neurological disorder caused by damage to the portions of the brain that are responsible for language production or processing. This is an impairment of language, It may occur suddenly or progressively, depending on the type and location of brain tissue involved. Primary signs of the disorder include difficulty in expressing oneself when speaking, trouble understanding speech, and difficulty with reading and writing. Aphasia is not a disease, but a symptom of brain damage. Aphasia is always due to injury to the brain-most commonly from a stroke, particularly in older individuals. But brain injuries resulting in aphasia may also arise from head trauma, from brain tumors, or from infections. The disorder doesn't affect your intelligence, but does impair your ability to process language, read, write and talk.

AVM: stands for Arteriovenous Malformation. An AVM is a tangle of abnormal and poorly formed blood vessels (arteries and veins). They have a higher rate of bleeding than normal vessels. AVMs can occur anywhere in the body

Cerebral Angiogram: is a minimally invasive medical test that uses x-rays and an iodine-containing contrast material to produce pictures of blood vessels in the brain. In cerebral angiography, a thin plastic tube called a catheter is inserted into an artery in the leg through a small incision in the skin.

Chiropractic Functional Neurology: Chiropractic Neurologists are highly trained and qualified experts of the brain, spine and nervous system. As in medicine, the chiropractic profession has specialists who serve their community's patients, as well as providing expert evaluations and consultation to other physicians and health care practitioners

Circle of WIllis: circle of vessels found above the base of the brain where most aneurysms are found

Clipping: is a way to treat an aneurysm by placing a small metal clip across the neck of the aneurysm-the base of the bulge. The aneurysm is thereby sealed off from the blood flow; it cannot burst or spill blood into the brain.

Coiling: Once the catheter reaches the aneurysm, a very thin platinum wire is inserted. The wire coils up as it enters the aneurysm and is then detached. Multiple coils are packed inside the dome to block normal blood flow from entering. Over time, a clot forms inside the aneurysm, effectively removing the risk of aneurysm rupture. Coils remain inside the aneurysm permanently. Coils are made of platinum and other materials, and come in a variety of shapes, sizes, and coatings that promote clotting.

Craniotomy: A craniotomy is a surgical operation in which a bone flap is temporarily removed from the skull to access the brain

Endovascular Embolization: your doctor inserts a long, thin tube (catheter) into a leg artery and threads it through blood vessels to your brain using X-ray imaging. Your surgeon positions the catheter in one of the feeding arteries to the AVM, and injects an immobilizing agent, such as small particles or a glue-like substance, to block the artery and reduce blood flow into the AVM.

Flooding: Many brain injury victims experience sensory overload of the brain by: sounds; light and feeling. to be touched, move, or to be moved, vibrations; odor (sense of smell); own thoughts; etc ...Sensory over stimulation or 'Flooding' occurs after brain injury because the brain's 'filters' no longer work properly. It is an exhaustive situation if more pieces of information or stimuli are received than the brain can handle. A stimulus is information that we perceive through our senses; see, hear, smell, taste, touch (external stimuli) or through our mind or our body / proprioception (internal stimuli).

Functional plasticity: The brain's ability to move functions from a damaged area of the brain to other undamaged areas.

Gamma knife: is a non-invasive stereotactic radiosurgery instrument that involves no scalpel or incision – it's not a knife at all. Instead, the Gamma Knife uses up to 201 precisely focused beams of radiation to control malignant and nonmalignant tumors, as well as vascular and functional disorders in the brain, without harming surrounding tissues

Hemorrhagic Stroke: caused by (bleeds)

Ischemic stroke: caused by (clots)

MRA: stands for Magnetic resonance angiography–also called a magnetic resonance angiogram or MRA–is a type of MRI that looks specifically at the body's blood vessels. Unlike a traditional angiogram, which requires inserting a catheter into the body, magnetic resonance angiography is a far less invasive and less painful test.

MRI: Magnetic resonance imaging (MRI) is a test that uses powerful magnets, radio waves, and a computer to make detailed pictures inside your body. Your doctor can use this test to diagnose you or to see how well you've responded to treatment. Unlike X-rays and CT scans, an MRI doesn't use radiation. MRI lets doctors see very detailed images of the inside of your body. MRI passes through bone and takes pictures of soft tissue, such as tendons, blood vessels. During MRI or MRA, in some cases, a special dye, known as a contrast dye is used to improve the clarity of the images or pictures of your body's internal structures. This may be added to your bloodstream to make your blood vessels easier to see. When needed, the contrast is given with an intravenous (IV) needle.

SAH: Abbreviation for subarachnoid hemorrhage (SAH) is a life-threatening type of stroke caused by bleeding into the space surrounding the brain. SAH can be caused by a ruptured aneurysm, AVM, or head injury.

Structural plasticity: The brain's ability to actually change its physical structure as a result of learning.

Vestibular system: sensory system that is essential to normal movement and equilibrium.

Acknowledgements

There are so many people that I need to thank for their time and dedication. This book would not exist without them. It takes a team to accomplish a project like this and I know I would not have been able to finish without their support. So, a huge THANK YOU to…

My husband, Billy McIntyre; my sister, Laurie Jameson; my mom, Carol Schigg; the staff and editors at Author Academy Elite; Judy Belk; Lisa Habig; Paula Norton; Alta Thompson; and Katy Tuck.

About the Author

Sheri McIntyre is a first-time author. She is a wife and mother who lives south of Boston. On January 1, 2016, Sheri sustained a life-threatening brain hemorrhage. From the time Sheri started recuperating and could barely articulate her words, she expressed the desire to write a book. She wants to help others who may be going through medical issues that are life changing. Sheri wants to inspire and educate others about brain injury and compel others to THINK.

How I am now - As I write this, three years have passed. Since my life changed from the AVM rupture (brain hemorrhage) the world doesn't just stop and adapt. I realize that I have to choose to be in it or not. So, I choose to live my life every day! As I lay in bed in the morning, I wake up feeling, "normal." It's when I start moving around when things start feeling differently or become difficult. I guess I'm learning to adapt to the challenges that I am living with. I try to see the good in the bad and move through it. Knowing that some things will pass. The one thing I can count on is change! I never say never because I don't know what tomorrow will bring. Good or bad I deal with it and move on. There is just so much to do in a day and it can get very overwhelming; but I prioritize and do what I can!

I exercise now; which I never did! And I realize how beneficial it has become to my well-being and growth. I try to eat healthy and to do the right thing. As for the brain AVM - it's gone. So, I remain doing the best I can with what I have! I'm still dizzy-ish constantly, balance issues, speech, and forgetfulness all plague me. Flooding and over stimulation also are a part of my daily life. Some of these symptoms are getting better, but another MRI showed that my right cerebellum has been destroyed. So, despite the challenges I keep moving forward!

Grateful and Very Blessed!
THINK,
Sheri

CONTACT SHERI

My website http://sherithink.com/

Made in United States
North Haven, CT
24 May 2022

19495737R00059